Diagnostic Tests and Procedures

Applying the Nursing Process

Diagnostic Tests and Procedures

Applying the Nursing Process

Zara R. Brenner, R.N., M.S.
Assistant Professor of Nursing
State University College at Brockport
Brockport, New York

APPLETON & LANGE
Norwalk, Connecticut/Los Altos, California

0-8385-1594-0

Notice: Our knowledge in clinical sciences is constantly changing. As new information becomes available, changes in treatment and in the use of drugs become necessary. The author(s) and the publisher of this volume have taken care to make certain that the doses of drugs and schedules of treatment are correct and compatible with the standards generally accepted at the time of publication. The reader is advised to consult carefully the instruction and information material included in the package insert of each drug or therapeutic agent before administration. This advice is especially important when using new or infrequently used drugs.

87 88 89 90 91 / 10 9 8 7 6 5 4 3 2 1

Prentice-Hall of Australia, Pty. Ltd., Sydney
Prentice-Hall Canada, Inc.
Prentice-Hall Hispanoamericana, S.A., Mexico
Prentice-Hall of India Private Limited, New Delhi
Prentice-Hall International (UK) Limited, London
Prentice-Hall of Japan, Inc., Tokyo
Prentice-Hall of Southeast Asia (Pte.) Ltd., Singapore
Whitehall Books Ltd., Wellington, New Zealand
Editora Prentice-Hall do Brasil Ltda., Rio de Janeiro

Library of Congress Cataloging-in-Publication Data

Brenner, Zara R.
Diagnostic tests and procedures.

Bibliography: p.
Includes index.
1. Diagnosis, Laboratory. 2. Nursing. I. Title.
[DNLM: 1. Diagnosis, Laboratory—nurses' instruction.
2. Diagnostic Tests, Routine—nurses' instructions.
3. Nursing Assessment—methods. 4. Nursing Process—methods. WY 100 B838d]
RT48.5.B74 1987 616.07'5 87-1311
ISBN 0-8385-1594-0

Production Editor: Elizabeth Ryan
Design: Cindy Lee Lombardo
Cover: Steve M. Byrum

PRINTED IN THE UNITED STATES OF AMERICA

To my husband, Charles Mitchell Brenner,
for being all that he is.

Contents

Preface xi

Acknowledgments xiii

Introduction xv

1. The Technology of Diagnostic Procedures 1
- Ultrasonography 1
- Magnetic Resonance Imaging 4
- Scintigraphy 4
- Radiology 5
- Computed Tomography 6
- Contrast Studies 8
- Biopsy 11

2. Clients with Alteration in Tissue Perfusion 13
- Laboratory Tests 15
- Electrocardiography 21
- Phonocardiography and Phonoangiography 27
- Ultrasonography 28
- Plethysmography 31
- Magnetic Resonance Imaging 34
- Scintigraphy 35
- Radiology 45

Computed Tomography 46
Lumbar Sympathetic Block 48
Contrast Studies 50
Renin Studies 56

3. Clients with Potential for Injury or Infection 59
Laboratory Tests 60
Ultrasonography 69
Scintigraphy 70
Lymphangiography 73
Bone Marrow Biopsy, Bone Marrow Aspiration 75

4. Clients with Impaired Gas Exchange 77
Laboratory Tests 79
Skin Testing 82
Pulmonary Function Tests 86
Ultrasonography 90
Magnetic Resonance Imaging 91
Scintigraphy 92
Radiology 95
Computed Tomography 98
Contrast Studies 100
Direct Visualization 104
Biopsy 106

5. Clients with Alterations in Nutrition, Metabolism, and Elimination 109
Laboratory Tests 111
Gastric Analysis, Diagnex Blue 120
Motility and Challenge Tests 122
Breath Tests 131
Ultrasonography 134
Magnetic Resonance Imaging 136
Scintigraphy 138
Radiology 149
Computed Tomography 151
Contrast Studies 153
Direct Visualization 160
Biopsy 166

6. Clients with Impaired Fluid Volume 169
Laboratory Tests 171
Ultrasonography 175

Magnetic Resonance Imaging 177
Urodynamic Measurements 178
Scintigraphy 181
Radiology 185
Computed Tomography 186
Contrast Studies 188
Direct Visualization 196
Percutaneous Renal Biopsy 199

7. **Clients with Impaired Mobility** **201**

Laboratory Tests 202
Ultrasonography 205
Ocular Plethysmography 207
Measurement of Electrical Activity 209
Thermography 212
Magnetic Resonance Imaging 213
Scintigraphy 215
Radiology 222
Computed Tomography 224
Direct Visualization 226
Biopsy 228
Spinal Puncture 233
Contrast Studies 241

8. **Clients with Alterations in Sensory Input** **247**

Tests for Sensory Acuity 248
Direct Visualization 253
Tonometry 256
Measurement of Electrical Activity 257
Ultrasonography 260
Radiology 261
Fluorescein Angiography 262
Caloric Stimulation Test 263

9. **Clients with Sexual Dysfunction** **265**

Laboratory Tests 267
Ultrasonography 271
Magnetic Resonance Imaging 273
Radiology 274
Computed Tomography 276
Direct Visualization 278
Biopsy 282

10. Clients with Potential Alteration in Family Process **285**

Fertility Tests 286
Contrast Studies 290
Fetal Testing 292
Prenatal Testing 294

References 299

Index 305

Preface

This book was developed in response to my awareness of a recurring discrepancy: after undergoing a diagnostic procedure, clients and friends would report that they did not expect what actually happened. Yet years of working with nurses show that nurses do conscientiously teach clients before diagnostic procedures. The discrepancy arises because many nurses have not seen the procedures, and while they know—and teach—the purpose of the test, they do not know and cannot teach specifically what happens to the client during the procedure.

Some of the diagnostic procedures discussed in this book may be performed with minimal specific nursing input. Yet clients are holistic beings, needing health care from many different disciplines. In order for nursing care to be most beneficial, nurses must incorporate knowledge from the other disciplines in their treatment of their clients.

The organization of this book stems from my avid support of the use of nursing diagnoses as the organizational framework of the profession. Every attempt has been made to apply the results of the Seventh National Conference on Nursing Diagnosis. It was noted at the Conference that other diagnoses merit consideration for acceptance in the future, thus acknowledging that other nursing diagnoses may yet be needed. Some clinical situations discussed in this text required diagnoses to be formulated.

Acknowledgments

Thank you to my friends and colleagues for their encouragement and assistance. To Patricia Fennell, R.N. for providing support and information when I needed both; to Drs. Robert Spitzer, Theodore Van Zandt and Paul Weiss for providing the illustrations in Chapter 1; to Ann Moy and Marion Kalstein-Welch for their editorial guidance.

I also want to thank my parents, Aubrey and Amelia Jay, and my children, Stacey Ellen and Melissa Sloane, for helping me to keep going and get done.

Introduction

The framework of this book is the use of nursing diagnoses and the nursing process. Each section is headed by a broad nursing diagnosis and includes the procedures that a client with that nursing diagnosis may undergo. The procedures are, for the most part, arranged by degree of invasiveness, progressing from noninvasive to invasive. Specific nursing diagnoses and the nursing process are applied to clients undergoing each procedure.

Many tests provide data that are important to more than one nursing diagnosis. For this resaon, many procedures and nursing diagnoses overlap. An attempt has been made to place each procedure according to its major, or one of its major outcomes. To avoid repetition, each test is listed only once. Therefore, it may be necessary to use the index to locate some procedures, especially laboratory tests.

Many diagnostic procedures performed today constitute little physical risk to the client in and of themselves, so postprocedure physical evaluation of the client is minimal. The author feels strongly, however, that while the physical impact on the client may be minimal, each test does impact on the psyches of the client and family. Thus, while specific nursing evaluation of the client's physical status may be minimal or nonexistent, clients still require emotional support following a procedure, especially if testing is related to a specific complaint or suspected disease.

In using this book, the reader should keep in mind several points. The laboratory values listed are guidelines. Individual laboratory results vary widely, and the reader must obtain the normal values from the laboratory performing the test. There is also much variation in the physical preparation of clients for diagnostic procedures. The client preparation in this book serves as a general guideline. The reader is reminded to confirm any specific client preparation with the department performing the test. Chapter 1 explains the technology currently available. It is recommended that the reader first refer to the appropriate section of Chapter 1 before reading the individual procedure.

Diagnostic Tests and Procedures

Applying the Nursing Process

1

The Technology of Diagnostic Procedures

This section explains the technology of various diagnostic techniques. Examples of the resulting imaging are included to help the user understand how the results are interpreted and applied to each client.

ULTRASONOGRAPHY

Ultrasound is a noninvasive procedure that can be performed anywhere and involves minimal client preparation or discomfort. Ultrasound uses sound waves in the range of 1–15 MHz, above human hearing, directed at body structures. Tissues of different composition reflect sound waves at different intervals allowing for ultrasonic diagnosis of boundaries between the tissues. A boundary with air reflects back almost all sound, making ultrasound ineffective. Figures 1–1A and 1–1B show examples of normal and abnormal ultrasound images.

Air must be excluded between the transducer and the client. Thus, gel is placed on the client and the transducer is moved along the skin with some pressure. For soft areas that move when pressure is applied, i.e., the breasts or male genitalia, a water bath scanner is used. The desired part of the client is surrounded by a contained water solution while the scanner moves along the container.

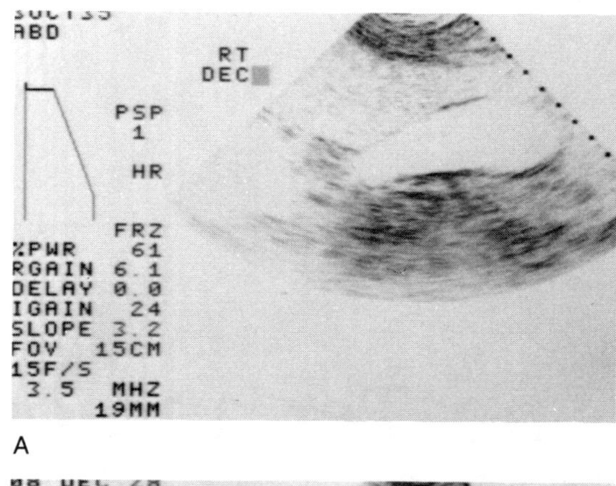

A

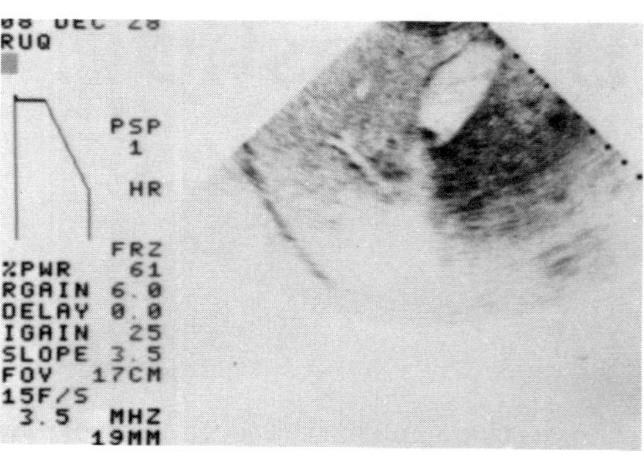

B

Figure 1–1. A. Ultrasound demonstrating normal gall bladder. **B.** Ultrasound of gall bladder demonstrating gall stone.

Several different display modes are used for ultrasonography, either singly or in combination. *A mode* or *A scan* displays are vertical lines indicating the amplitude of the echo. *B mode, B scan,* or *2D* results in a two-dimensional display of dots that vary in brightness in correlation with the echo intensity. With the use of digital scan convertors, data regarding echo amplitude arising from within organs and structures can be stored and updated. Different scanners may be used in B mode. Static B scanners use a moving probe and continuous recordings of the display to result in a cross-sectional image. Real-time scanners produce sequential image frames fast enough to follow changes in spatial relationships occurring within the anatomical plane, i.e., valve movement, etc.

M mode, also a brightness display, uses a moving recording surface to display data about rapidly occurring events. "Real-time" ultrasonography uses sweeping motion across the client's chest to provide a fan-shaped picture of moving parts of the body, i.e., cardiac valves.

Doppler ultrasonography is based on the Doppler effect that states that blood flow velocity is proportional to the difference in frequency be-

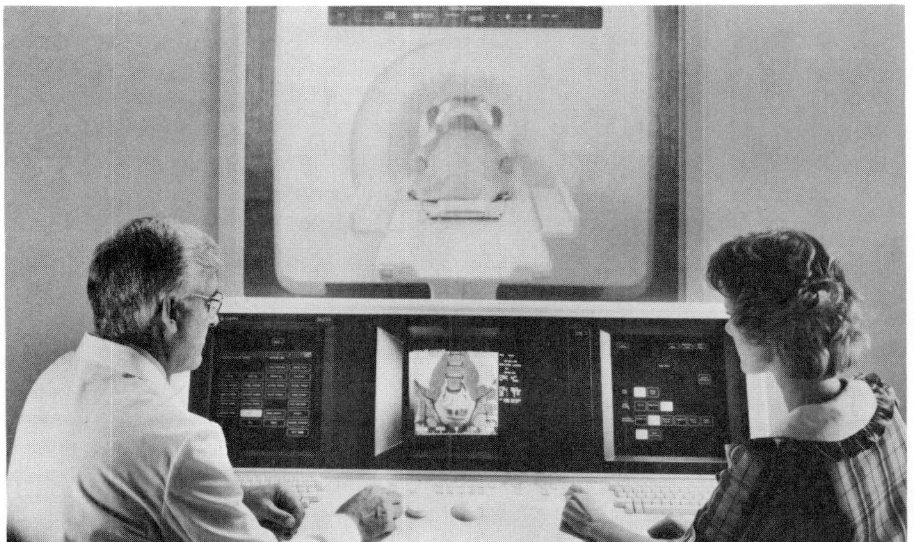

A

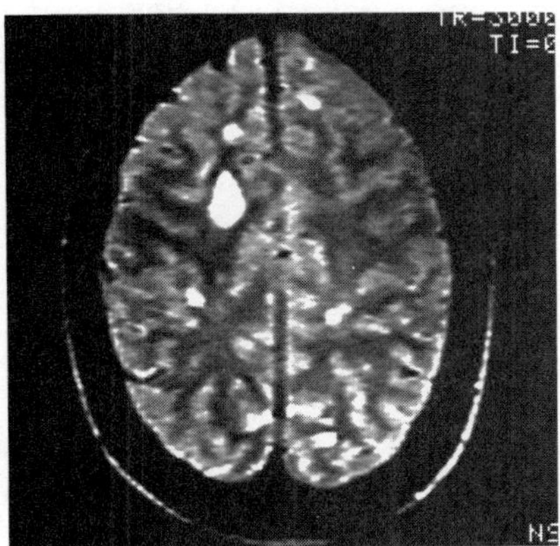

B

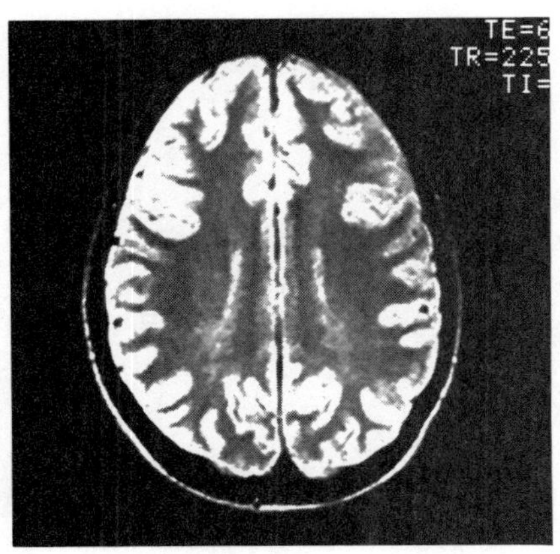

C

Figure 1–2. A. The Signa Magnetic Resonance Imager system's multitasking capability lets one operator conduct a scan while another operator reviews images from previous studies. (Courtesy General Electric Company, Medical Systems Group, Milwaukee Wisconsin.) **B.** Normal MRI of the brain. **C.** MRI of the brain demonstrating the presence of multiple sclerosis lesions.

tween the sound transmitted toward and reflected from a vessel containing a moving stream of blood. Continuous-wave Dopplers detect only blood flow velocity. Pulsed Dopplers detect blood flow at a desired, specific distance from the probe by blocking some receiver gates so that more rapid, i.e., closer, echoes are not amplified. Doppler probes are small, hand-held devices.

MAGNETIC RESONANCE IMAGING (NUCLEAR MAGNETIC IMAGING, MR, NMR)

Magnetic resonance imaging is a noninvasive method of assessing tissue function and chemical composition. A magnetic resonance imager (MRI) is shown in Figure 1–2. MRI results in three-dimensional computerized imaging of proton movement within the hydrogen atoms in the body. (Figs. 1–2B and C). After placing the body area to be studied in a machine-created magnetic field, the energy state of the protons is raised. As the excited protons move back to their original positions, they emit energy that is transmitted as radiofrequency. The computer records each proton's radiofrequency energy emission as a dot and composes an image using those dots. The completed imaging can appear in either gray scale or full color. Small variations in tissue physiochemistry cause visible differences in MR signals.

MRI is considered to have several advantages when compared with computed tomography (CT). Ionizing radiation is not involved. MRI requires a relatively short imaging time. MRI appears to be a superior technique for determining the chemical composition of tissues within the body. MRI is contraindicated for clients with aneurysm clips or pacemakers due the use of the magnetic field. At the present time, there are no known risks associated with MRI.

SCINTIGRAPHY (NUCLEAR MEDICINE)

Except for an injection, scintigraphy is a noninvasive technique that provides data on anatomic and physiologic activity within the body. A small amount of organ-specific radiopharmaceutical is either taken orally or injected intravenously. When the radioisotope concentrates in the desired area, imaging with a gamma camera takes place (Figs. 1–3A and B). The readings are fed to a computer that produces interpretive data about function and also constructs images.

Scintigraphy has many advantages and is widely used to obtain data about physiology. Adverse reactions to the procedure are rare, since the

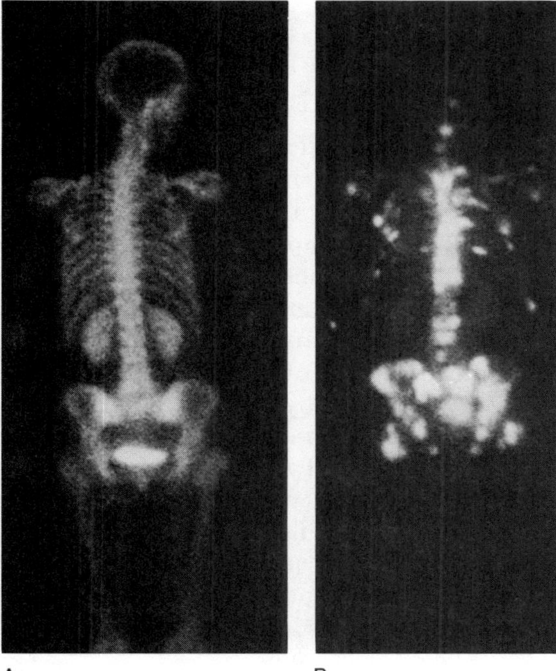

Figure 1–3. A. Normal bone scan. **B.** Bone scan demonstrating bone metastasis.

quantity of radiopharmaceutical injected is so small. The half-lives of the radioisotopes are short, resulting in minimal exposure for the client or others. The amount of radioactivity is minute. Imaging can be repeated several times, in most instances without the need for additional injections of radioisotopes.

Blocking agents, nonradioactive substances, may be needed to prevent organs other than the one being studied from taking up the radioisotope. Blocking agents are most commonly used in conjunction with iodine-tagged radioisotopes. Lugol's solution will protect the thyroid from iodine-tagged radiopharmaceuticals. Clients who are allergic to iodine will receive potassium perchlorate to protect the brain. Pregnancy and lactation are contraindications to scintigraphy.

RADIOLOGY

Radiology is based on the ability of roentgen rays (x-rays) to penetrate tissues or organs differently according to tissue density and thickness. As the waves pass through and are absorbed by the tissues, images in varying degrees of dark and light are formed on photographic film behind the client. The greater the energy absorbed, the whiter the image appears on film. Bones, calcium deposits, surgical wires, etc., are whitest, whereas air-filled space is blackest.

Radiography has established its value over many years of use. The concern with radiography is the cumulative effect of ionizing radiation exposure. Ionizing radiation "ionizes" atoms or molecules, thereby altering their chemical behavior. In sufficient quantities, ionizing radiation destroys cells. At this point in time it is impossible to determine a threshold below which damage can be guaranteed not to occur. The National Academy of Science's Advisory Committee on Radiation has recommended that the general population be limited to 170 mrem of exposure per person per year. Specific quantities of radiation exposure per exam are difficult to state as they are affected by the specific machinery used, the length of exposure, and the skill of the radiology team. Radiology exams should be performed only when specifically indicated. Lead shields are applied to surrounding body areas to protect the client against unnecessary exposure. Personnel working with radiographic devices should protect themselves. Radiation devices must be carefully monitored to provide maximum client benefit and minimum client risk. New "dedicated," use-specific, radiologic machinery requiring less ionizing radiation to produce a sharp image is constantly being developed.

Tomography is radiographic imaging through a predetermined cross section of the body. Overlying structures are blurred so that areas otherwise concealed can be examined.

COMPUTED TOMOGRAPHY (CT SCAN, CT, EMI)

Computed Tomography uses ionizing radiation, but in a different way from conventional radiography. For CT, a radiation detector rather than photographic film is used. Multiple narrow x-ray beams are used as the x-ray tube and radiation detector rotate around the client (Fig 1–4A). The radiation detector is connected to a computer that analyzes the readings and, via mathematical formulas, calculates the amount of radiation absorbed and constructs a three-dimensional transverse image (Figs 1–4B and C). The computer can also analyze the data to measure tissue density and can reconstruct the images in different planes, i.e., sagittal and coronal planes. For contrast-enhanced CT scanning, the client receives contrast medium in order to further delineate certain structures.

CT has proved to be advantageous. It provides much of the data, especially regarding the central nervous system, that were previously obtainable only by invasive procedures. Scatter radiation is limited, so that each exposure receives only its own ionizing radiation.

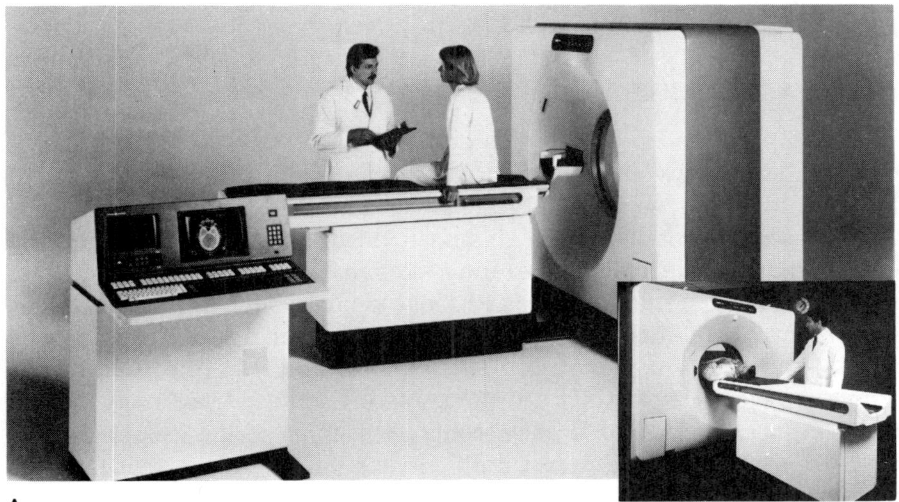

A

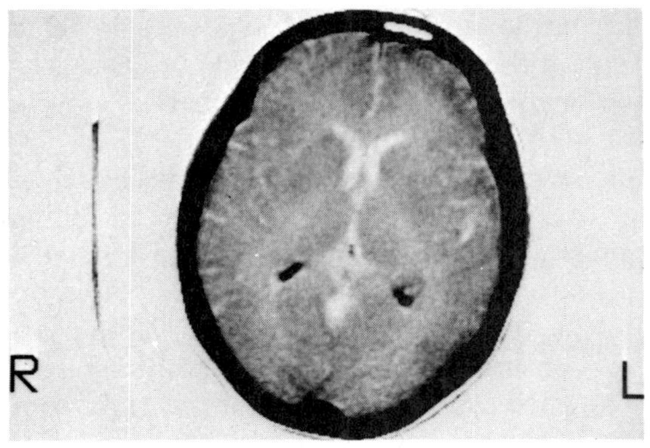

B

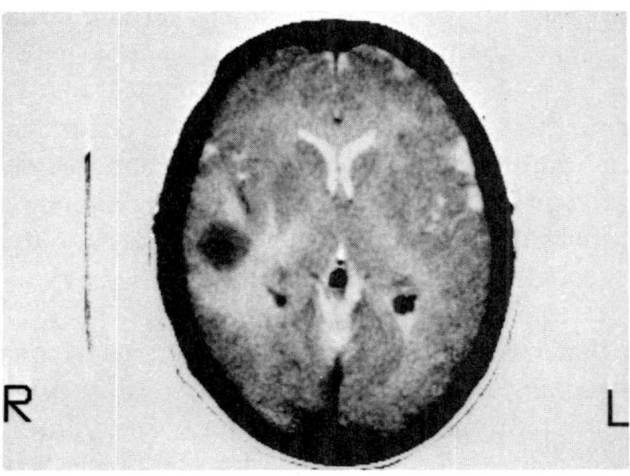

C

Figure 1–4. A. The General Electric CT 9800 Quick computed tomography system combines an advanced x-ray scanning system with a powerful computer to permit study of virtually any portion of the human anatomy. *(Courtesy of General Electric Company, Medical Systems Group, Milwaukee, Wisconsin.)* **B.** Normal CT scan of the brain. **C.** CT of the brain demonstrating presence of a tumor.

CONTRAST STUDIES

Contrast studies involve the insertion of a contrast medium into the client followed by timed, serial radiographs. Because fluoroscopy and/or serial radiographs are involved, the client's exposure to ionizing radiation is higher than with a single radiographic examination. The contrast medium may be a "dye," a radiographically dense medium such as barium, or air. Depending on the body part to be examined, contrast medium may be administered by intravenous (IV) or intra-arterial (IA) injection, orally, via various gastrointestinal tubes, via the bronchii, intraspinally, or rectally. Figures 1-5A and B show contrast studies of the esophagus.

For intravascular contrast studies, reaction to the contrast medium is a constant concern. There are three types of client reactions.

"Minor" reactions occur in approximately 5% of clients. This consists of nausea, vomiting, bradycardia, and transient hypotension. This type of reaction usually occurs within minutes of injection and lasts less than 1 hour. Clients are NPO prior to contrast studies to prevent aspiration should this reaction occur.

"Allergic" or anaphylactoid reactions occur in approximately 2% of clients. Which clients will have this response cannot be predicted. Signs range from urticaria and wheezing to sustained hypotension and laryngeal edema. Clients with a previous history of allergic response are tested by intradermal (ID) injection of a test dose of contrast medium. If no reaction occurs, the full dose of IV contrast medium is then administered. Medication can reduce the recurrence rate of this type of reaction from 30% to 5% for clients who need further testing. Steroid therapy (prednisone 50 mg) is begun 18 hours prior to examination and antihistamine therapy, diphenhydramine HCl (Benadryl 50 mg) is administered 1 hour prior to injection. A specific informed consent dealing with the issue of allergic reaction is obtained.

"Vasomotor collapse" or "contrast-induced renal failure" occurs in approximately 0.15% of clients. Oliguria and rising serum creatinine levels occur within 48 hours of administration of the contrast medium. They are usually transient. The mean duration of oliguria is 2–4 days. Adequate client hydration prior to the procedure may play a major role in preventing this reaction.

In addition to the risk associated with contrast medium reactions, the impact on the client of vascular contrast studies is affected by type of vessel punctured and catheter manipulation within the vessel. Thus, IV puncture and contrast medium insertion via a peripheral vein carries relatively little risk to the client and is easily performed on an outpatient basis. Arterial puncture and catheter manipulation to a selected vessel imposes a greater risk. Complications are rare but may include hemor-

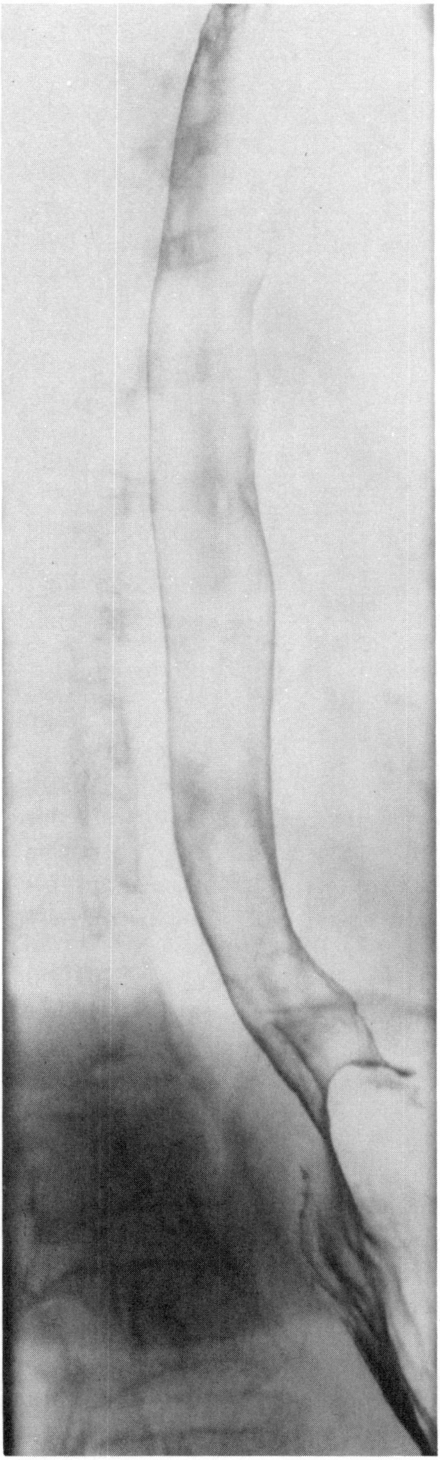

A

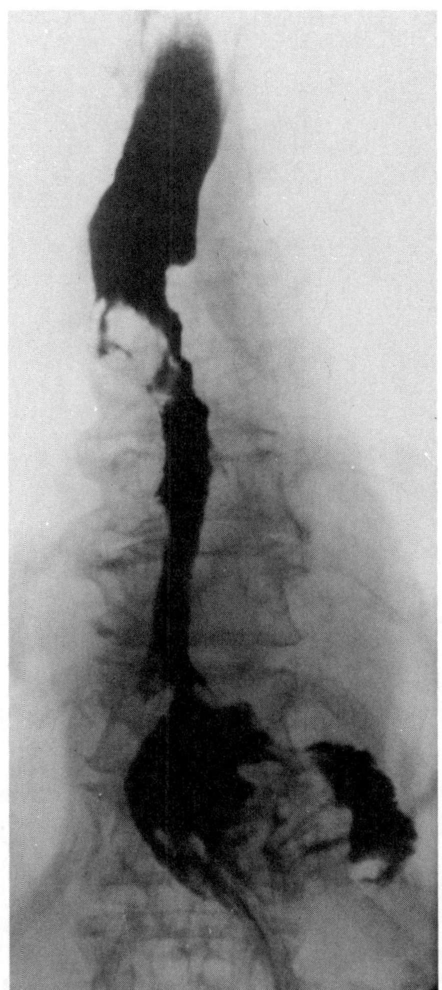

B

Figure 1–5. **A.** Double contrast of normal esophagus. **B.** Single contrast study demonstrating stenosis of the esophagus.

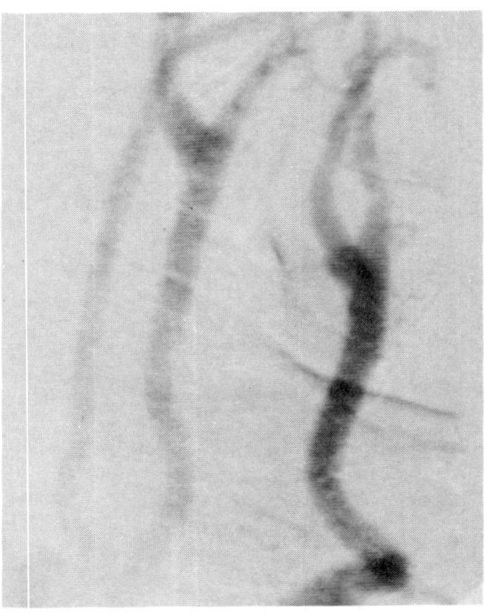

A

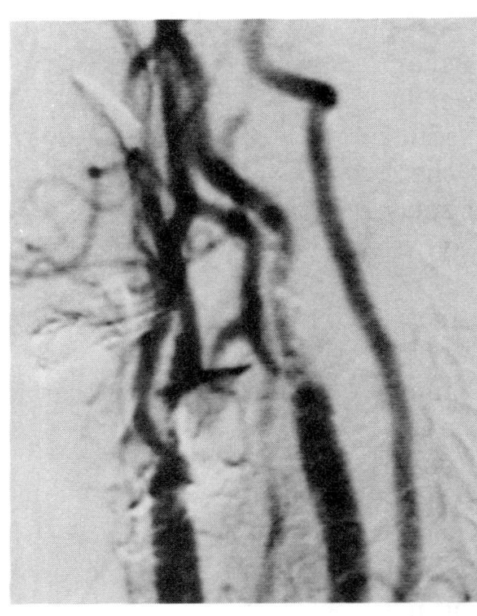

B

Figure 1–6. A. Normal DSA of carotid and vertebral arteries. **B.** DSA demonstrating occluded internal carotid artery and vertebral artery stenosis.

rhage, vessel damage, and embolization with its attendant risks. Postprocedure monitoring is required to ensure that the client safely recovers from the procedure. This may affect the feasibility of outpatient testing for some clients. The increased resources, time, space, and personnel, contribute to make intraarterial angiography a more expensive procedure.

Digital subtraction angiography (DSA) (Figs. 1-6A and B) is an image enhancement system that amplifies low concentrations of intravascular iodine in order to obtain data concerning malfunctions in the heart or aortic, carotid, renal, or femoral arterial systems. Fluoroscopic images of the desired area are obtained. Following administration of contrast material, the area is again imaged. The computer subtracts the initial image, the "mask," from second, "mask mode subtraction," resulting in an image of an isolated iodine-containing structure. Thus, the computer provides data on the desired heart chamber or blood vessel free from interference of overlying soft tissue or bone. DSA is obtained by itself, or in conjunction with contrast studies such as intravenous pyelogram or cardiac catheterization. DSA may be performed using venous (IV DSA), arterial (IA DSA), or intracoronary injection.

DSA has several advantages when compared with conventional angiography. IA DSA requires approximately one-third less contrast material. This means smaller and softer catheters can be used that decrease both local and distal complications secondary to catheter manipulation and placement. IA DSA thus lends itself more readily to outpatient use. IV DSA also uses smaller catheters and lower doses of contrast medium and reduces the need for vessel selective catheterization and catheter manipulation. This is especially advantageous for clients with suspected carotid artery disease or those with tortuous vessels. Additionally, DSA is less expensive.

DSA does have limitations. Movement during imaging significantly affects the quality of the mask. If the client cannot cooperate, the results may be ineffective for diagnosis. Cardiac output must be sufficient to administer the contrast medium in a bolus to the desired area. Although the amount of contrast medium is less, the quantity of fluid given the client during DSA is significant. Serum BUN and creatinine levels must be adequate prior to the procedure.

For gastrointestinal tract contrast studies, the contrast medium is inserted directly into the GI tract. Risks secondary to the contrast medium and its administration are less than those associated with intravascular contrast studies. Client impact may still be high and depends on the client's reaction to administration of the contrast medium. Potential complications include postprocedure impaction and perforation of the GI tract if any tubes are used to insert the contrast medium.

BIOPSY

Many pathophysiologies require biopsy for definitive diagnosis. Several methods exist for removing a tissue portion for analysis. Biopsies are obtained from the skin's surface and from within the body via a scope or percutaneous puncture. Specimens are analyzed by a variety of microscopic and/or laboratory techniques. Biopsies are invasive, although the degree of client involvement depends on the structure being biopsied and its location within the body.

2

Clients with Alteration in Tissue Perfusion

Clients with alterations in tissue perfusion are cared for by nurses in all clinical settings. These clients range in age from newborns to the elderly. Disease affecting the cardiovascular system is the most common health problem in our country. Clients with impaired tissue perfusion undergo repeated diagnostic testing in order to assess and monitor their cardiovascular status. Clients with alterations in tissue perfusion face tremendous physiologic and psychologic impact. Nursing diagnoses during care address psychosocial needs and pathophysiologic concerns.

Physical examination is the first step in assessing clients with impaired tissue perfusion. A thorough personal history, family history, and history of the present illness are obtained. A detailed record is taken of the client's subjective complaints. The physical examination itself is extensive and reflects each individual client's status.

Inspection, palpation, percussion, and auscultation are used to assess the heart, its valves, rate, and rhythm. Examination of the arterial system includes assessing the presence and quality of all pulses. Blood pressure is recorded as a ratio, in millimeters of mercury (mm Hg), of the pressure needed to expel blood through the arteries during systole (contraction phase) to the pressure needed to expel blood through the arteries during diastole (relaxation phase). Blood pressure may be measured in different sites and/or positions. Cuff size is important and is correlated to client size, i.e., adult, obese adult, child, etc. Physical examination of the venous system includes assessing jugular vein pulsations (JVP). Assessment of veins may include bilateral measurements of the extremities. In addition, the following tests may be performed.

Although not specific for deep vein thrombosis, Homan's sign is frequently used as an assessment tool. It consists of sharp dorsiflexion of the foot and is considered positive when associated with calf pain.

The Brodie–Trendelenburg test is used to assess superficial vein valve competence in clients with suspected varicose veins. The client is supine, with the affected leg raised to empty the veins. A tourniquet is then applied to the upper thigh and the client stands. Superficial vein filling is assessed before and after the tourniquet is removed.

The Perthes' test uses a tourniquet to assess the deeper and communicating veins. After a tourniquet has been placed just below the knee, the client is instructed to walk. Lack of emptying and distension upon walking imply deep venous incompetence or obstruction.

LABORATORY TESTS

Clients with alterations in tissue perfusion often undergo multiple laboratory procedures. Client education is essential since many tests require specific timing, preparation, or other client involvement to be accurate. Inadequate client knowledge is costly in terms of time, efficiency, and money.

Nursing Diagnoses for clients undergoing laboratory tests include:

- Anxiety related to procedure
- Knowledge deficit related to diagnostic process

LABORATORY TESTS

Test	Purpose	Normal Values	Nursing Actions
CPK isoenzymes Serum	Assess myocardial damage	CPK: total Female: <51 mU/ml Male: <82 mU/ml CPK-MB (CPK 2): indicates cardiac damage CPK-MM: indicates skeletal muscle damage	Usually done on a serial basis, i.e., × 3 days
Erythrocyte fragility Serum	Assess anemia	Hemolysis begins at 0.45–0.39% Hemolysis ends at 0.33–0.30% saline solution	
Erythroprotein Serum	Assess anemias, renal disease	7–36 mille immunochemical units/ml	
Ferritin Serum	Assess hematopoietic status	Adult female: 5–100 ng/ml Adult male: 10–270 ng/ml	
Folic acid Serum	Assess anemias	4–16 ng/ml	

(Continued)

LABORATORY TESTS (cont.)

Test	Purpose	Normal Values	Nursing Actions
Glucose-6-phosphate dehydrogenase deficiency test (GPD, G-6PD) Serum	Assess hemolytic anemia or deficiency	Varies with lab	
Glutathione reductase (GR) Serum	Assess anemia	9–13 U/g Hgb	
Heinz bodies Serum	Assess anemia	Negative	
Hemoglobin electrophoresis Serum	Assess types and structure of hemoglobin; diagnose Thalassemia	HgA: 96.5%–98.2% HgA2: 1.8%–3.5% HgF: Adult: 0% Infant: 2%–10% Newborn 40%–70% Albumin: 3.5–5.5 g/100 ml A1 globulin: 0.1–0.4 g/100 ml A2 globulin: 0.1–1.0 g/100 ml Beta globulin: 0.5–1.1 g/100 ml Gamma globulin: 0.5–1.7 g/100 ml	Determine if client has had blood transfusion within 4 mo, as this may affect results
Iron Serum	Assess anemias	Adult: 87–279 3–10 yr: 53–119 6 wk–3 yr: 20–115 Newborn: 20–157	
Total iron binding capacity (TIBC)	Assess amount of iron that could be carried if transferrin were completely saturated	3 yr to adult: 250–400 Newborn to 3 yr: 59–175	
Percent saturtion	Assess current level	3 yr to adult: 20–55 6 wk–3 yr: 10–55 Newborn: 65	

Test	Purpose	Normal Values	Nursing Actions
Lipids total Serum	Assess this risk factor	400–1000 mg/100 ml	Client is NPO 12 hrs prior to test
Cholesterol	Assess hepatic, pancreatic, biliary tract, thyroid function, xanthomatosis	40 yr +: 150–300 mg/dl 30–39 yr: 140–270 mg/100 ml 20–29 yr: 120–240 mg/100 ml 1–19 yr: 120–230 mg/100 ml Newborn: 50–120 mg/100 ml HDL: Female: 35–80 mg/100 ml Male: 30–65 mg/100 ml LDL: 60–190 mg/100 ml VLDL: 25–50%	
Triglycerides	Assess hepatic, thyroid function, diabetes mellitus	Older adult: 20–200 mg/100 ml Adult: 20–150 mg/100 ml	
Phospholipids		130–380 mg/100 ml	
LDH isoenzymes Serum	Assess myocardial damage: positive when LDH1>LDH2	LDH_1: 25%–33% LDH_2: 35%–41% LDH_3: 16%–22% LDH_4: 6%–10% LDH_5: 3%–7%	Usually done on a serial basis, i.e., × 3
Potassium Serum	Determine level	3.5–5.0 mEq/L	Monitor for clients receiving diuretic or potassium therapy
Red blood cells (RBC) (Part of a CBC)	Assess for anemias, hydration, oxygen transport	Older adult: 3–5 mil/cu mm Adult female: 4.2–5.5 mil/cu mm Adult male: 4.4–6.0 mil/cu mm Child after age 2: same as adult	Do not draw from same extremity as IV infusion

(Continued)

LABORATORY TESTS (cont.)

Test	Purpose	Normal Values	Nursing Actions
RBC (cont.)		Newborn: 3.5–8.2 mil/cu mm	
Hematocrit (HCT) (packed red cell volume)	Assess blood loss, hydration, hematologic disorders	Adult female: 37%–47% Adult male: 42%–52% Child: 31%–43% Infant: 30%–40% Newborn: 44%–64%	Do not draw from same extremity as IV infusion
Microhematocrit (Fingerstick)		Adult female: 42%–44% Adult male: 45%–47% Child: 35%–39% Newborn: 56%	
Hemoglobin (Hgb)	Assess blood loss, anemias, dehydration, heavy lead intoxication	Adult female: 12–16 g/100 ml Adult male: 14–18 g/100 ml Child: 11.2–13.4 g/100 ml Infant: 10–15 g/100 ml Newborn: 12.2–20 g/100 ml	
Hgb S	Diagnose sickle cell anemia	Negative	May be inaccurate if Hgb is <10 g/100 ml in infants under 6 mo
RBC indices	Assess anemias and polycythemia		
Mean corpuscular hemoglobin (MCH)		Older adult: 28–32 pg Adult: 27–34 pg Child: 27–31 pg Newborn: 32–34 pg	
Mean corpuscular hemoglobin concentration (MCHC)		Older adult: 29%–33% Adult: 30%–40% Child: 32%–36% Newborn: 32%–33%	

Test	Purpose	Normal Values	Nursing Actions
Mean corpuscular volume (MCV)		Older adult: 90.5–105.5 cu μg Adult: 82–101 cu μg Child: 82–97 cu μg Newborn: 96–108 cu μg	
Reticulocyte count Serum	Assess anemia, chronic disease	Adult female: 0.5%–1.5% Adult male: 0.5%–2.5% Child: 0.5%–4% Infant: 2%–5% of total erythrocytes	
Vitamin B_{12} Serum	Assess anemia	200–1100 pg/ml	Client is NPO overnight prior to test

Please note, these values are guidelines. Check with the laboratory performing the procedure for absolute values.

DRUG LEVELS

Drug	Effective Concentrations	Nursing Actions
Captopril	50 ng/ml	
Diazoxide	35 μg/ml	
Digoxin	0.8–2 ng/ml	Draw before dose or 6 hours after to avoid misleading fluctuations in level
Digitoxin	10–30 ng/ml	
Disopyramide	>3 μg/ml	
Hydralazine	100 ng/ml	
Labetolol	0.13 μg/ml	
Lidocaine	Therapeutic: 1.4–6 μg/ml Toxic: >10 μg/ml	Do not draw from same extremity as IV infusion
Lorcainide	40–200 ng/ml	
Metoprolol	25 ng/ml	
Mexiletine	Therapeutic: 0.7–2.0 μg/ml Toxic: >2.0 μg/ml	
Nitroglycerin	1.2–11 ng/ml	

(Continued)

DRUG LEVELS (cont.)

Drug	Effective Concentrations	Nursing Actions
Pindolol	58 ng/ml	
Procainamide	2–12 μg/ml	
Propanolol	20 ng/ml	
Quinidine	2–6 μg/ml	
Timolol	15 ng/ml	
Tocainide	6–15 μg/ml	
Verapamil	100 ng/100 ml	

Please note, these values are guidelines. Check with the laboratory performing the procedure for absolute values.

ELECTROCARDIOGRAPHY

- **12 Lead**
- **Holter Monitoring**
- **Exercise Testing**
- **Electrophysiology Studies**

Electrocardiography (ECG) records electrical activity within the heart. ECG interpretation is a major tool in the diagnosis and treatment of clients with cardiac disease. It is also used for routine screening. A specific consent form is required for Stress Testing and Electrophysiology Studies.

Nursing Diagnoses for clients undergoing electrocardiography include:

- Anxiety related to procedure
- Potential alteration in cardiac output related to activity during the procedure
- Knowledge deficit related to diagnostic process

12 Lead (Standard, Resting, ECG [EKG])

Subjective Data: Client complains of pain, dizziness, syncope, palpitations, "feeling one's heart beat," and fatigue.

Objective Data: Client may be asymptomatic; this may be the first procedure in the diagnostic process, or the client may present with rhythm disturbances or hypotension.

Assessment: This procedure may be part of a routine check-up or a vital monitoring mechanism for the client with known cardiac disease. It provides data on the initiation of impulses, transmission of impulses within the heart, and the axis (rotation) of the heart within the body. Twelve different leads are recorded, including the bipolar limb leads, I, II, and III; the augmented unipolar limb leads, AVR, AVL, and AVF; and six precordial (chest) leads, V_1–V_6. Right precordial leads, V_{1R}–V_{6R}, may be obtained to detect the presence of right ventricular infarction. Effects of chemical activity such as electrolyte imbalance or drug therapy on cardiac function can also be evaluated. Computers are used to record, store, retrieve, and interpret ECGs.

Nursing Interventions: Clients need to be directed to lie still during the procedure to avoid voluntary muscular activity from interfering with the recording. Nurses frequently perform this procedure.

Description of the Procedure: The procedure can be performed wherever there is an ECG machine. The client reclines during this procedure. Privacy is assured. For a one-time screening procedure, shaving even a hirsute client is probably unnecessary. On an inpatient acute care unit however, small areas on the chest and extremities may be shaved. If a client has lost a limb, the electrodes are placed bilaterally equidistant from the heart. A small dab of conductive gel or cream is placed on each of the client's extremities and on six locations on the chest. The electrodes are wrapped securely on the extremities. To obtain the six precordial leads, the bell-shaped electrode is placed in each of the following positions:

Standard precordial leads:

- V_1—fourth intercostal space at the right sternal border
- V_2—fourth intercostal space at the left sternal border
- V_3—midway between V_2 and V_4
- V_4—fifth intercostal space at the mid-clavicular line
- V_5—horizontal to V_4 at the anterior axillary line
- V_6—horizontal to V_4 at the mid-axillary line

Right precordial leads:

- V_{1R}—fourth intercostal space at the left sternal border
- V_{2R}—fourth intercostal space at the right sternal border
- V_{3R}—midway between V_2 and V_4
- V_{4R}—fifth intercostal space at the right mid-clavicular line
- V_{5R}—horizontal to V_4 at the right anterior axillary line
- V_{6R}—horizontal to V_4 at the right mid-axillary line

Computerized ECGs use six chest leads placed simultaneously. A "minute strip," a continuous recording for 1 minute in a preselected lead, may also be recorded. The electrodes and gel are removed. This procedure is completed in less than 5 minutes. The tracing can be immediately interpreted by appropriate personnel.

Evaluating Client Response: For nonscreening ECGs, the results may be the basis for immediate client treatment; thus, appropriate nursing actions are implemented. Client and family support is provided as needed.

■ Holter Monitoring (Avionics)

Subjective Data: Client complains of dizziness, weakness, syncope.

Objective Data: The presence of known or suspected cardiac dysrhythmias, postcardiac surgical status or anti/arrhythmic drug therapy.

Assessment: Holter monitoring provides a continuous record of the client's heartbeat for 12 or 24 hours. A magnetic tape records the client's cardiac rhythm. The tape is scanned and changes in rhythm are correlated with changes in time and activity. Thus, episodic symptoms and drug response can be studied.

Nursing Interventions: Client education includes an explanation of the procedure. Specific instructions are provided regarding not disturbing the electrodes. Showering or bathing during the test is not permitted. The activity form and the importance of returning on time for completion of the test are explained. During avionics, the nurse provides assistance, as needed, as the client completes the activity form.

Description of the Procedure: This procedure is performed with inpatients and outpatients. Electrodes are attached to the client's chest in the usual manner and then taped so that they remain secure for the time period ordered. The avionics recorder is in a carry case that the client wears over the shoulder or on a belt. Frequently, the client is given an activity form and asked to record activities and symptoms that occur during the test period. The results are available after scanning and interpretation by a cardiologist.

Evaluating Client Response: Client and family support is provided.

■ Exercise Testing (Exercise Tolerance Test (ETT), Stress Test)

Subjective Data: Client complains of pain.

Objective Data: Findings are equivocal on physical examination or standard ECG, or as an evaluation of medical or surgical therapy.

Assessment: This procedure monitors electrical activity within the heart as the cardiac workload is increased. Exercise testing provides an accurate description of how cardiac disease affects the heart's ability to meet the body's demands for oxygen and deal with relative ischemia. This procedure is used to assess the presence of ischemic cardiac disease, degree of cardiac impairment caused by existing disease, response to various medical therapeutic regimens, postsurgical and/or predischarge exercise status, and exercise program capability and appropriateness. Exercise testing is performed on an individualized basis or "protocol." This prescription for how much and how quickly exercise can be attempted is based on factors including age, sex, physiologic status, medications, physical fitness, and the reason for the test. The test is considered positive if and when the client reports chest pain, or with the onset of ST depression of 1 mm or more, arrhythmia, hypotension, inappropriate tachycardia, or an S3. This procedure is also used in conjunction with Thallium testing. (See the section on thallium testing in this chapter.)

Nursing Interventions: Client education includes an explanation of the procedure. Clients are encouraged to be well-rested and are not allowed to smoke, eat, or drink for 4 hours before the test. Medication administration prior to the test is determined on a individual basis. Clients are told to bring comfortable walking shoes and appropriate underwear to the test. The importance of telling the tester of any new or different sensations that occur during the test, such as pain, discomfort, pressure, etc. is emphasized. Consideration is given to scheduling this procedure so that there is adequate client rest time before and after. Some laboratories request that clients bring their own nitroglycerin tablets with them, others do not. A complete, current medication record should accompany both inpatients and outpatients.

Description of the Procedure: This procedure is performed with inpatients and outpatients. In addition to the equipment required for the exercise test, emergency drugs, equipment, and personnel are present in case a client experiences an adverse response to the exercise-induced increased cardiac workload. The procedure begins with baseline measurement of the ECG, blood pressure, and respiratory rate. The client then starts walking on the treadmill slowly and at a slight incline. The treadmill is periodically speeded up and the incline raised. The client's ECG is continuously monitored and periodic blood pressure readings are obtained. The client is asked for subjective comments. An exercise tolerance test is completed when the client finishes the protocol or if the test is positive as described above. Postexercise ECG, blood pressure, and respiratory rate are recorded. If there has been any adverse response, the client stays in the lab until cardiac status returns to baseline. This procedure is completed in less than 1 hour. The results are available as soon as interpreted by the cardiologist.

Evaluating Client Response: In the event of a positive test, monitoring of cardiovascular status, i.e., vital signs and ECG, continues until the client's baseline status is achieved. Food and medications are resumed. Positive exercise tests are frequently the basis for further testing and/or medical intervention. Client and family support is provided.

■ Electrophysiology Studies (EPS, Cardiac Mapping)

Subjective Data: Client complains of fatigue, dizziness, or syncope.

Objective Data: Abnormal ECG indicating the presence of dysrhythmia, or a history of unexplained syncopal episodes.

Assessment: This procedure combines regular surface ECGs with intracardiac electrocardiography and pacing. EPS is used to identify the mechanism of an arrhythmia to determine the cause of syncope, to identify clients at high risk for lethal ventricular arrhythmias, to assess the response to drug therapy, and to determine the need for mechanical pacing and/or surgery. By stimulating different parts of the conduction system, its response and any resulting dysrhythmias can be studied in detail. When a dysrhythmia is induced, it may require treatment to resolve, including drug therapy, cardioversion, or short term anesthesia.

Nursing Interventions: Client education includes an explanation of the procedure. The client is told that the procedure is designed to elicit arrhythmias so that they can be assessed. The client is reassured that the laboratory has the personnel and equipment to treat any arrhythmias. The client is NPO prior to the procedure, overnight if the test is scheduled for the morning, or after a clear liquid breakfast when an afternoon time is scheduled. The client voids prior to the procedure.

Description of the Procedure: This procedure is usually performed with inpatients. The client goes to the EP laboratory. The entry site, usually the femoral, internal jugular, or subclavian vein is located and prepared. More than one entry site may be used. Catheters are inserted into the vein(s) and threaded via fluoroscopy to the heart. Occasionally, a catheter may be inserted via the femoral artery. Baseline surface and intracardiac ECGs are recorded and compared. Various parts of the conduction system are stimulated according to client need. Mapping, the process of locating the site of origin of a recurrent ventricular tachycardia may also be undertaken. The client's status is stabilized before the client leaves the EP laboratory. This procedure is completed in 3–4 hours. Occasionally, a catheter may be left in place for followup studies the next day. The results are available upon completion of the procedure.

Evaluating Client Response: Vital signs and insertion sites are monitored every 15 minutes the first hour, every 30 minutes for the next hour, and every hour thereafter prn. Clients are on bed rest with the insertion site immobilized for 2 hours after a venous entry or for 12 hours after an arterial entry. A pressure dressing or sandbag may be applied to an arterial site. Food and medications are resumed. Specific additional monitoring may be needed appropriate to any medication the client received during the procedure. Telemetry monitoring may also be needed depending on the arrhythmias elicited. If a catheter has been left in place, special positioning and sterile dressing changes may be required. Client and family support is provided.

PHONOCARDIOGRAPHY AND PHONOANGIOGRAPHY

These procedures provide a graphic recording of heart and arterial sounds respectively. No specific consent form is required.

Nursing Diagnoses for clients undergoing phonocardiography or phonoangiography include:

- Anxiety related to procedure
- Knowledge deficit related to diagnostic process

Subjective Data: Client complains of pain, dizziness, syncope, fatigue, or palpitations.

Objective Data: Altered physical findings include murmurs, clicks, rubs, or bruits.

Assessment: These procedures are performed to assess clients with suspected valvular disease or arterial occlusion. Since these tests pose no risk to the client, they are frequently the first diagnostic procedures performed following physical examination.

Nursing Interventions: Nursing actions include preprocedure client education.

Description of the Procedure: These procedures are performed with inpatients and outpatients and may be performed bedside for acutely ill clients. The client reclines comfortably. To promote optimal sound transmission, conductive gel or cream is placed on the surface above the area to be examined. The transducer, attached to the graphic recorder, is placed on the client and moved across the skin to obtain a complete recording. Clients may be asked to change positions during the procedure. The procedure is completed in less than 30 minutes. The results are available after interpretation.

Evaluating Client Response: Postprocedure client and family support is provided.

ULTRASONOGRAPHY

- **Echocardiography**
- **Peripheral Ultrasonography**
- **Doppler Examination**

Structure and blood flow through the heart and blood vessels can be delineated by analyzing sound waves aimed at those structures and the returning sound wave pattern. Ultrasonography is highly informative, noninvasive, and, therefore, widely used. No specific consent form is required for these procedures.

Nursing Diagnoses for clients undergoing ultrasonography include:

- Anxiety related to procedure
- Knowledge deficit related to diagnostic process

Echocardiography

Subjective Data: Client complains of chest pain, palpitations, or shortness of breath.

Objective Data: Altered physical examination including murmurs, rubs, and decreased heart sounds.

Assessment: This procedure is used to assess clients with congenital, ischemic, or acquired heart disease. Structure and mobility of the heart, each valve, and the pericardial sac are examined. Several different methods are used for display depending on the data desired.

Nursing Interventions: Client education includes an explanation of the procedure. Specific instructions include remaining still and feeling some pressure during the procedure.

Description of the Procedure: This procedure is performed with inpatients and outpatients. Portable units allow bedside use. For echocardiography, the client reclines comfortably and remains still. Privacy is assured. To ensure optimal contact between transducer and skin, conductive oil or gel is placed on the client's chest. The transducer is moved across the precordium according to the cardiac structures that need examining. The client may be aware of pressure being applied to the transducer. This procedure takes approximately 30–45 minutes. The results are available following interpretation.

Evaluating Client Response: Client and family support is provided.

■ Peripheral Ultrasonography

Subjective Data: Client complains of pain, tingling sensations, or numbness.

Objective Data: Altered physical examination includes poor or absent pulses, bruits, and skin and nail changes.

Assessment: Ultrasound is used to examine morphologic features of the abdominal aorta and lower extremity peripheral arterial vessels. It is rapid, noninvasive, and demonstrates the true size of the vessel. B mode ultrasonography is the definitive diagnostic tool for assessing abdominal aortic aneurysms. Static B scanning is used for evaluating femoral, popliteal, and iliac vessels. Peripheral ultrasound is often used in combination with pulsed Doppler. (See the section on Doppler examination.)

Nursing Interventions: Client education includes an explanation of the procedure and specific instructions regarding remaining still during the procedure.

Description of the Procedure: This procedure is performed with inpatients and outpatients and can be done bedside. The client is positioned according to the area to be studied. Conductive oil or gel is placed on the skin to allow for optimal contact with the transducer. The transducer is moved across the skin according to the area to be studied. Several views, thus, several positions, may be required. Palpation of the vessel may accompany ultrasound examination. This procedure is completed in less than 30 minutes. The results are available following interpretation.

Evaluating Client Response: Postprocedure support for client and family is provided.

■ Doppler Examination (Continuous Wave Doppler, Pulsed Doppler, Doppler Imaging)

Subjective Data: Client complains of dizziness, syncope, pain, or altered peripheral sensations.

Objective Data: Altered physical examination including the absence of pulses, the presence of bruits, changes in skin and nail color, or altered response to peripheral stimuli.

Assessment: The Doppler blood flow detector is a small, hand-held device containing both transmitting and receiving crystals. Sound waves are directed at a blood vessel and the returning sound waves are amplified and can be recorded. Continuous Wave Dopplers detect blood flow beneath the skin. Pulsed Dopplers detect blood flow at a specific distance from the probe and are used for deeper peripheral vessels. Doppler imaging combines a Doppler probe, a position sensing arm and an oscilloscope for a visual image of a blood vessel. Dopplers are used to locate and assess non-palpable pulses as well as to accurately define the characteristics of a specific artery.

Nursing Interventions: Client education includes an explanation of the procedure and specific instructions regarding remaining still during the procedure. Nurses frequently use Dopplers.

Description of the Procedure: This procedure can be performed anywhere, due to the portability of the Doppler flow meter. The blood vessel to be examined is located. A small amount of conductive gel or cream is applied to the skin. The Doppler is moved slowly, proximally, and distally on the skin above that vessel with the examiner using anatomical direction and the audible beeping of the Doppler as guides. Comparisons may be made with other blood vessels. This procedure takes several minutes, according to the extent of the Doppler examination. The results are available immediately.

Evaluating Client Response: Client and family support is provided.

PLETHYSMOGRAPHY

- **Strain Gauge Plethysmography**
- **Impedance Plethysmography**
- **Photoplethysmography**

Plethysmography records peripheral vascular volume changes in response to externally applied pressure. Response is evaluated in terms of volume and time, thus providing data on vessel patency. Plethysmography is frequently used in conjunction with Doppler examination. No specific consent form is required.

Nursing Diagnoses for clients undergoing plethysmography include:

- Anxiety related to procedure
- Knowledge deficit related to diagnostic process

Strain Gauge Plethysmography

Subjective Data: Client complains of swelling, pain, intermittent claudication, tingling sensations, coldness, or numbness.

Objective Data: Altered physical findings including edema, skin changes, decreased or absent pulses, positive Homan's sign, or decreased sensitivity to peripheral stimuli.

Assessment: This procedure measures and records arterial inflow and changes in venous volume, maximum venous outflow (MVO), and wave fluctuation during respiration or valsalva maneuver in the extremities.

Nursing Interventions: Client education includes an explanation of the procedure and specific instructions regarding maintaining the required position.

Description of the Procedure: This procedure is performed with inpatients and outpatients and may take place in a vascular laboratory or may be performed bedside. Client position is dependent on the area being examined. To assess the lower extremities, for example, the client is supine with head flat, feet elevated, knees bent, and the hip externally rotated to keep pressure off the calf and popliteal vein. A blood pressure cuff is applied to the thigh and monitoring leads placed distally. The cuff is inflated to the level of venous pressure, approximately 50 mm Hg, to occlude venous outflow. Increases in volume distal to the cuff represent the rate of arterial inflow. The plethysmograph tracing is used to determine maximal calf vein distension. When that point is reached, occlusive thigh cuff pressure is released and the MVO recorded. A delayed MVO indicates the presense of thrombosis. This procedure is completed in one-half hour. The results are available following interpretation.

Evaluating Client Response: Postprocedure care includes client and family support.

■ Impedance Plethysmography (IPG)

Subjective Data: Client complains of swelling or pain.

Objective Data: Altered physical findings including edema, skin changes, or positive Homan's sign.

Assessment: This procedure is sensitive and specific for proximal vein thrombosis involving the popliteal, superficial femoral, common femoral, external iliac, and common iliac veins. This method is based upon the principle that relates blood volume changes to changes in electrical resistance (impedance).

Nursing Interventions: Client education includes an explanation of the procedure and specific instructions regarding maintaining the required position.

Description of the Procedure: This procedure is performed with inpatients and outpatients and may be performed bedside or in a vascular laboratory. Client position is dependent on the extremity being examined. To assess a lower limb, for example, the client assumes a supine position with the leg elevated, knee flexed 10–20 degrees and ankle slightly higher than the knee. A pneumatic cuff is applied at midthigh and electrodes are placed distally surrounding the calf. The midthigh cuff is inflated to occlude venous return. After a predetermined period of time (45–120 seconds), cuff pressure is released suddenly and the changes in electrical resistance distal to the cuff are recorded by ECG machine. This procedure is completed in less than 30 minutes. Results are available following interpretation.

Evaluating Client Response: Postprocedure client and family support is provided.

■ Photoplethysmography (Photoelectric Plethysmography, PPG)

Subjective Data: Client complains of swelling, pain, numbness or tingling.

Objective Data: Altered physical findings including skin changes.

Assessment: This technique uses infrared light and the microcirculation of the skin. A probe transmits infrared light toward the skin while recording reflected light by means of an infrared-sensitive phototransistor attached to an amplifier. When clients with impaired peripheral vascular circulation exercise, vascular response is less than normal and returns to baseline faster. PPG is also used to assess the internal carotid artery system.

Nursing Interventions: Client education includes an explanation of the procedure and specific instructions as to exercise during the procedure.

Description of the Procedure: This procedure is performed with inpatients and outpatients. The client goes to the vascular laboratory, where room temperature and extraneous light are controlled. At the start, a baseline measurement is obtained, for example, of the ankle, when leg circulation is being evaluated. The client exercises by dorsal and plantar flexion of the foot. Measurements are taken at the culmination of exercise and until the preexercise level is reached. Mean venous recovery time is 48 seconds for clients with normal circulation but is significantly shorter for clients with peripheral vascular disease. To assess the internal carotid artery system, the probe is placed on the forehead or other area supplied by the frontal and supraorbital arteries. The examiner applies pressure to occlude the circulation and records recovery. This procedure is completed in 30 minutes. Results are available following interpretation.

Evaluating Client Response: Postprocedure client and family support is provided.

MAGNETIC RESONANCE IMAGING, (NUCLEAR MAGNETIC IMAGING, MR, NMR)

MR is a noninvasive method of assessing tissue composition. A specific consent form may be required.

Nursing Diagnoses for clients undergoing MR include:

- Anxiety related to procedure
- Knowledge deficit related to diagnostic process

Subjective Data: Client complains of pain and altered sensations in the extremities.

Objective Data: Altered physical findings and abnormal data from prior diagnostic procedures.

Assessment: The use of MR to determine function and chemical tissue composition of the heart is under investigation. Difficulties exist in gating respirations in order to examine the thorax. MR has been shown to be more effective for assessing clients with suspected vascular disease. MR is contraindicated in clients with aneurysm clips anywhere in the body, or with pacemakers because of the effects of the magnetic field.

Nursing Interventions: Client education includes an explanation of the procedure and the need to remain still during the imaging. The ability of the child to cooperate by lying still is determined. Sedation and restraints are usually required for infants and small children. A client's health history specific to past insertion of aneurysm clips or pacemaker is obtained. Clients are prepared for the imposing size of the MR scanner, whereas the noninvasive nature of the procedure is emphasized. The client changes into a hospital gown, removes all jewelry and prostheses.

Description of the Procedure: This procedure is performed with inpatients and outpatients. In the MR room, the client lies supine within the body scanner. MR imaging is completed in less than 30 minutes. Results are available after interpretation.

Evaluating Client Response: Postprocedure client and family support is provided.

SCINTIGRAPHY

- Perfusion Imaging
- Infarct Imaging
- Nuclear Angiocardiography
- Radionuclide Angiography
- Iodine-125–Fibrinogen Uptake Test
- Iodine-125–Fibrinogen Leg Scintigraphy
- Radionuclide Venography
- In Vivo Studies
- Schilling Test

Several different scintigraphic studies are used to assess clients with impaired tissue perfusion. Scintigraphic procedures are noninvasive, and thus precede and are preferred, when possible, to contrast studies. The development of the portable gamma camera allows imaging at the bedside. A specific consent form may be required for these procedures.

Nursing Diagnoses for clients undergoing scintigraphy include:

- Anxiety related to procedure
- Knowledge deficit related to diagnostic process

Perfusion Imaging (Thallium Scanning, Cold Spot Scanning)

Subjective Data: Client complains of chest pain, dyspnea, or fatigue.

Objective Data: Dysrhythmias, hypertension, shortness of breath, edema, or equivocal findings on other diagnostic procedures.

Assessment: Normally, thallium-201 (Tl-201) distributes evenly throughout the myocardium. Thus, deficits in thallium uptake identify areas of myocardial fibrosis and ischemia. Quantitative graphic results can also be obtained. Perfusion imaging at rest is considered very sensitive in detecting myocardial infarction, especially during the initial phase when other indicators are not yet definitive or ECG interpretation is questionable. A major use of thallium scanning is in combination with exercise testing. (See the section on electrocardiography.) Thallium exercise testing is used when routine exercise tests are equivocal or when angiography has shown stenosis with questionable physiologic effect. Scintigraphy is contraindicated during pregnancy and lactation.

Nursing Interventions: Client education includes an explanation of the procedure. Prior to a thallium exercise scan, clients are told to bring comfortable clothes and shoes. The importance of telling the tester immediately if any adverse sensations occur is emphasized. The client is prepared for the waiting period between the two imaging times and the possible insertion of an IV line. Scheduling considerations include separating different nuclear medicine studies by 24–48 hours to reduce potential cross interference. Beta-blocking pharmacotherapy may be reduced prior to thallium exercise testing to reduce the likelihood of false negative results. If this therapy is reduced, additional client monitoring is required. Clients may be restricted to clear liquids for 4–8 hours prior to this test. Arrangements are needed for client safety and comfort during the time lapse between the first and second imaging.

Description of the Procedure: This procedure is performed with inpatients and outpatients. Resting perfusion imaging can be done bedside with a mobile camera. For thallium exercise testing, the client goes to the designated area. Baseline ECG and vital signs are recorded. An IV line may be inserted. The client then exercises to 1 minute short of peak. Electrocardiographic stability is determined and a single injection of Tl-210 is given intravenously. The client exercises to peak and is then positioned under the scintillation camera. Three or four different views that require camera and client repositioning are taken. Four hours later, the imaging process is repeated. This procedure encompasses approximately 5 hours, including the waiting period. The results are available following interpretation.

Evaluating Client Response: Postprocedure support for client and family is provided.

■ Infarct Imaging (Myocardial Imaging, Technetium Scanning, Hot Spot Imaging)

Subjective Data: Client complains of chest pain, dyspnea, or fatigue.

Objective Data: Dysrhythmias, hypertension, shortness of breath, edema, or equivocal findings on other diagnostic procedures.

Assessment: This procedure uses a radiopharmaceutical, most commonly technetium-99m-pyrophosphate, that concentrates in damaged myocardium. This technique is used to diagnose myocardial infarction in clients whose ECG is already altered, such as postcoronary surgery clients. Infarct imaging is most accurate when performed at least 12 hours and within 1–3 days after the onset of suspected myocardial infarction. Scintigraphy is contraindicated during pregnancy and lactation.

Nursing Interventions: Client education includes an explanation of the procedure. Scheduling considerations include 24–48 hours between different nuclear medicine studies in order to reduce potential cross-interference.

Description of the Procedure: Infarct imaging is frequently used in the early postoperative period and as such may be done bedside in an intensive care unit. This procedure requires a single intravenous injection of radioactive tracer substance followed by positioning of the gamma camera above the client. The procedure takes approximately one-half hour. The results are available following interpretation.

Evaluating Client Response: Postprocedure care includes support for the client and family.

■ Nuclear Angiocardiography (Gated Blood Pool Studies, MUGA Scans, Gated Pool, Gated Wall Motion, Equilibrium Studies or First Pass, First Transit Studies)

Subjective Data: Client complains of chest pain, dyspnea, or fatigue.

Objective Data: Altered physical findings including shortness of breath, edema, or hypertension, and abnormal findings on other diagnostic procedures.

Assessment: Nuclear angiocardiography includes two different methods for evaluating anatomic and physiologic status of the heart. Gated blood pool studies i.e., the client's ECG triggers the imaging, are used to assess cardiac effectiveness. The relative size and structure of parts of the heart and quantitative measurement of cardiac activity and ventricular function are obtained. Indices of ventricular effectiveness, such as ejection fractions and ventricular volumes are determined by the computer. Visual evidence of anatomic structures and wall motion are obtained. First-pass studies are used to assess clients with lung disease, cardiomyopathy, wall motion abnormalities, shunts, or aneurysms. This technique uses the computer to record changes in radioactivity within the ventricle as a time-activity curve. End-systolic and end-diastolic blood volumes and ejection fractions are also determined. Scintigraphy is contraindicated during pregnancy and lactation.

Nursing Interventions: Client education includes an explanation of the procedure with specific instructions regarding positioning. Scheduling considerations include 24–48 hours between different nuclear medicine studies in order to reduce potential cross-interference. When acutely ill clients undergo gated blood pool studies, the time required for the procedure must be a consideration in planning nursing care such as medication administration.

Description of the Procedure: These procedures are performed with inpatients and outpatients and may be done bedside for acutely ill clients. The client is positioned according to the view to be obtained. Two IV injections, the first containing unlabeled pyrophosphate and the second containing Tc-99m-pertechnetate are administered. Imaging begins approximately 5 minutes later. Repeat injections of the radiopharmaceutical are required for first-pass studies but not for gated blood pool studies. First-pass studies require one view whereas gated blood pool studies require three or four views to obtain maximum data. For each view, the client is positioned and asked to maintain that position for approximately 10 minutes. Gated blood pool studies require approximately 1 hour, whereas first-pass studies require less than one-half hour. The results are available following interpretation.

Evaluating Client Response: Client and family support is provided following the procedure.

Radionuclide Angiography

Subjective Data: Client complains of pain, tingling, and other altered sensations.

Objective Data: Altered physical findings including bruits, skin color and temperature changes, and altered findings on prior diagnostic testing.

Assessment: Dynamic flow studies and static imaging are used to assess degree of arterial flow reduction, presence of collateral circulation or efficacy of surgical intervention. Large arteries, such as the iliac, femoral or subclavian, are visualized via static studies, whereas dynamic flow images are used to determine qualitative flow abnormalities in smaller vessels. Since other studies such as ultrasound, digital subtraction angiography, and computed tomography provide superior diagnostic results, radionuclide aortography is usually performed only in conjunction with other abdominal imaging. Scintigraphy is contraindicated during pregnancy and lactation.

Nursing Interventions: Client education includes an explanation of the procedure and specific instructions regarding positioning during imaging. Scheduling considerations include 24–48 hours between different scintigraphic procedures in order to reduce potential cross-interference.

Description of the Procedure: Radionuclide angiography is performed with inpatients and outpatients. The client is positioned according to the site of interest. The radiopharmaceutical is injected and imaging begun. Procedure time varies with the area being examined. Several views are taken to determine the extent of an aneurysm. Arteries are usually examined bilaterally and brachial artery examination requires two separate imagings because of field width limitations. For clients with Raynaud's phenomenon, imaging is used to record blood flow changes over several hours. The results are available following interpretation.

Evaluating Client Response: Postprocedure client and family support is provided.

■ Iodine-125–Fibrinogen Uptake Test, (I-125–FUT)

Subjective Data: Client complains of tenderness.

Objective Data: Altered physical findings including redness, tenderness, and increased temperature in the affected extremity or a positive Homan's sign.

Assessment: This procedure is used for clients with suspected thrombus formation in the deep veins. Sensitivity is highest in the calf veins. The results are stated in terms of a ratio of uptake at a leg location to uptake at the precordium. Scintigraphy is contraindicated during pregnancy and lactation.

Nursing Interventions: Client education includes an explanation of the procedure. A client history specific as to allergy to iodine is obtained.

Description of the Procedure: These clients are usually in the hospital for treatment, but the procedure can be performed anywhere. The client is supine in bed with privacy provided. Indelible ink marks are made every two inches from the inguinal ligament along the medial thigh distally to the ankle. A one-time IV injection of labeled fibrinogen is administered. This dose is sufficient for 1–2 weeks of client monitoring. Counts are taken that day, and every day until positive or for at least 7 days. Before each measurement, the client empties the bladder to avoid false high readings in the inguinal area and lies supine with legs elevated 15–20 degrees above the head for 5 minutes to promote venous emptying. The hand-held counter is then moved in sequence to each mark. A precordial reading is taken and serves as the 100% mark. Each scanning session takes less than 15 minutes. The results are available immediately.

Evaluating Client Response: Support for family and client is provided during the prolonged time period that this procedure is in use.

■ Iodine-125–Fibrinogen Leg Scintigraphy (Deep Vein Thrombosis Scan, DVT Scan)

Subjective Data: Client complains of tenderness.

Objective Data: Altered physical findings including redness, tenderness, and increased skin temperature in the affected extremity, or a positive Homan's sign.

Assessment: Iodine-125–fibrinogen leg scanning is used to confirm clinical evidence of venous thrombosis. This procedure is specific and sensitive for active thrombosis in calf veins and the lower half of the thigh. Whole body imaging is used to detect thrombophlebitis in the pelvic, femoral, or arm region. The injected I-125–fibrinogen concentrates in the forming clot, allowing for serial monitoring of clot size. Clinical trials are underway to determine if this method is effective in detecting deep vein thrombi in general surgical clients. Scintigraphy is contraindicated during pregnancy and lactation.

Nursing Interventions: Client education includes an explanation of the procedure plus an explanation that, during a time-limited period, imaging may be repeated without additional injection. A history specific as to allergy to iodine is obtained.

Description of the Procedure: This procedure can be performed with inpatients and outpatients. The client is positioned relative to the gamma camera. An injection of I-125–fibrinogen is administered intravenously. Images may be obtained at that time, although images taken 6–24 hours postinjection may be more clearly interpreted. The accumulation of I-125–fibrinogen continues for approximately 72 hours; thus, reinjection is not needed unless there is an even longer time lapse between views. This procedure takes less than 1 hour. Results are available following interpretation.

Evaluating Client Response: Postprocedure nursing includes client and family support. Treatment will begin immediately if the results are positive.

■ Radionuclide Venography

Subjective Data: Client complains of tenderness or pain.

Objective Data: Altered physical findings including redness, tenderness, edema, and increased skin temperature in the affected extremity, and abnormal findings from other diagnostic procedures.

Assessment: Lower extremity radionuclide venography is used to determine the source and extent of venous thrombosis in clients with documented, recurrent pulmonary embolism. Upper extremity radionuclide venography is used for clients with suspected abnormalities of the arm, allergy to contrast medium, or who are undergoing a perfusion lung scan. Scintigraphy is contraindicated during pregnancy and lactation.

Nursing Interventions: Client education includes an explanation of the procedure, with emphasis on positioning. Scheduling considerations include 24–48 hours between different scintigraphic procedures to reduce potential cross-interference.

Description of the Procedure: This procedure can be performed with inpatients and outpatients. The client lies supine on the imaging table. In leg venography, for example, two tourniquets are applied, one above the ankle and one below the knee. Injection of contrast medium is via the dorsal vessel of each foot. Following initial visualization on a scope, the ankle tourniquets are released and serial flow images of the calf and femoral vein are obtained. The knee tourniquets are then released and serial flow images of the thigh and pelvis are obtained. Additional images of the lower legs may be obtained. This procedure can be completed in less than 1 hour. Results are available following interpretation.

Evaluating Client Response: Postprocedure client and family support is provided.

■ In Vivo Studies

Subjective Data: Client complains of fatigue or pain.

Objective Data: Abnormal findings from a CBC and other abnormal physical findings such as pallor or jaundice, history positive for familial hemolytic anemia, drug reaction, or autoimmune disorder.

Assessment: These studies are used for clients with suspected anemias, particularly hemolytic anemias. They involve IV administration of a radioisotope followed by drawing of a blood sample for laboratory analysis. Scintigraphy is contraindicated during pregnancy and lactation.

Nursing Interventions: Client education includes an explanation of the procedure. The minute amount of radioactive tracer and its nonthreatening nature is emphasized. For those undergoing red cell survival tests (RCS), ongoing family and client support is provided and the importance of all blood samples is emphasized. Scheduling considerations include 24–48 hours between different nuclear medicine studies in order to reduce potential cross-interference. If clients are to receive iodinated tracer solution, a history specific to allergy to iodine is obtained.

Description of the Procedure: In vivo studies are performed with inpatients and outpatients.

Red Cell Mass: In the nuclear medicine department, 10 to 15 mm of the client's blood is drawn and mixed with the anticoagulant, Acid Citrate Dextrose. Chromium-51 is added to the vial. After 30 minutes at room temperature, all but a small amount kept for use as a standard, is administered intravenously to the client. Ten to 15 minutes later another blood sample is drawn and radioactivity of the sample measured. Red cell mass is calculated from the proportion of radioactivity of the tagged RBCs injected to radioactivity/ml of RBCs after mixing. This procedure takes approximately 1 hour. The results are available after interpretation.

Plasma Volume: In the nuclear medicine department, a solution of I-131 or I-128- albumin is injected intravenously into the client. A small amount is kept as a standard. After 15 minutes, a blood sample is drawn and the radioactivity of the sample is measured. Plasma volume is calculated from the proportion of radioactivity of the injected solution to radioactivity per milliliter of the plasma after mixing. The procedure takes approximately 30 minutes. The results are available after interpretation.

Total Blood Volume: This is usually calculated indirectly by adding the red cell mass and the plasma volume, but can also be measured directly by using tagged red blood cells and radioiodinated albumin. This requires injections as described above to first mix the tracer solution with the client's blood, return the solution to the client, and then obtain a sample for analysis. This procedure takes approximately 1 hour. The results are available following interpretation.

Red Cell Survival and Sequestration: This procedure is an ongoing process that measures the life span of red blood cells. Ten to 15 ml of the client's blood is withdrawn, and mixed with the anticoagulant Acid Citrate Dextrose. Cr-51 is then added to the mixture. After 30 minutes, the entire sample is returned intravenously to the client. Blood samples are drawn 3 times weekly for 2 weeks and twice per week for 2 more weeks. Red cell life span is calculated by using the known half-life normal red cells and the half-life of cells tagged with Cr-51. Concurrent monitoring over the spleen provides information on the role of the spleen in shortening red cell life. This procedure is not complete for approximately 1 month. Initial client preparation takes 1 hour. Follow-up blood sampling takes less than 15 minutes, but may be accompanied by external body scanning requiring another 15 or 20 minutes. The results are available following completion of the entire test.

Evaluating Client Response: Postprocedure care includes support for the client and family in dealing with the outcome. Pathology that is genetic in origin has a major impact on the entire family. Clients undergoing red cell survival testing require additional support to maintain cooperation over the long test period.

■ Schilling Test

Subjective Data: Client complains of fatigue or weakness.

Objective Data: Abnormal findings on physical examination including pallor and abnormal results from a CBC.

Assessment: The Schilling test is performed to determine the adequacy of the intrinsic factor, a component of gastric juice essential for absorption of vitamin B_{12}. Following oral ingestion of cobalt-57-labeled cyanocobalamin, the client receives an injection of nonradioactive vitamin B_{12}. This saturates the tissue binding sites. The client's 24-hour urine output is measured for radioactive vitamin B_{12}. Urinary excretion directly reflects absorption of orally administered vitamin B_{12}. Sometimes, intrinsic factor is added to the second injection. This addition has little effect on urinary excretion of radioactive vitamin B_{12} in clients with an absorption defect in the small intestine. Scintigraphy is contraindicated during pregnancy and lactation.

Nursing Interventions: Client education includes explanation of the procedure with specific instructions regarding the importance of cooperating in urine collection for the full 24 hours. Scheduling considerations include 24–48 hours between different nuclear medicine studies in order to reduce potential cross-interference. If needed, bone marrow examination must be performed prior to this test. Clients receive no parenteral vitamins for 3 days and no oral vitamins for 24 hours prior to this study. NPO status is maintained prior to the procedure and for the first 2 hours. Urine collection is strictly maintained for the entire 24-hour period. A catheter may be inserted if incontinence prevents accurate urine collection.

Description of the Procedure: This procedure is performed with inpatients and outpatients. The client is NPO after midnight prior to the test. The client drinks a small amount of solution composed of Co-57-labeled vitamin B_{12}. A 24-hour urine collection is started immediately. One hour later, the client receives an intramuscular injection of 1mg of nonradioactive vitamin B_{12}. The client is NPO for 2 more hours and then resumes a normal diet. At the end of 24 hours, the radioactivity of the client's urine is measured. The study may be repeated to test for small bowel absorption defect. The entire study period encompasses 24 hours, although after the intramuscular injection and the 2-hour NPO period, the client's only involvement is saving all urine. Results are available following interpretation.

Evaluating Client Response: Postprocedure care includes support for the client and family in dealing with the results. Food and medications are resumed.

RADIOLOGY

Chest x-rays provide data about general cardiac anatomy. No specific consent form is required.

Nursing Diagnoses for clients undergoing chest x-rays include:

- Anxiety related to procedure
- Knowledge deficit related to diagnostic process

Subjective Data: Client may be asymptomatic or complain of dyspnea.

Objective Data: Altered findings on physical examination.

Assessment: Chest x-rays provide data on cardiac position, the size of the chambers and great vessels, and calcification. They are frequently used as a routine screening procedure but are also used to follow a client's response to therapy, especially for clients with congestive heart failure. Chest x-rays are used to ascertain the location of monitoring catheters, pacemaker wires, etc. One or more views may be obtained.

Nursing Interventions: Nursing actions include an explanation of the procedure. The client wears a hospital gown and removes all jewelry.

Description of the Procedure: This procedure is performed with inpatients and outpatients and may be done bedside for acutely ill clients. Optimally, the client stands for this x-ray, but acutely ill clients can be positioned in bed. In order to provide optimal visualization, the client is asked to inspire and hold a deep breath. This test takes less than 10 minutes. The results are available following interpretation.

Evaluating Client Response: Postprocedure support is provided for client and family.

COMPUTED TOMOGRAPHY (CT, COMPUTERIZED AXIAL TOMOGRAPHY, CAT SCAN, EMI)

CT scanning of the heart and blood vessels has shown great potential for clinical use. A specific consent form is required.

Nursing Diagnoses for clients undergoing CT include:

- Anxiety related to procedure
- Knowledge deficit related to diagnostic procedure
- Potential for injury: allergic reaction related to procedure

Subjective Data: Client complains of pain or changes in endurance.

Objective Data: Altered physical findings and abnormal data from prior diagnostic procedures.

Assessment: CT is used to image the heart, major vessels, and vascular beds. CT is well-suited for diagnostic use in clients with coronary artery disease, pericardial disorder, and cardiac tumors. Ultrafast CT can be used for clients with valvular disease. Arterial CT scans can identify and measure aortic aneurysms, mural thrombii calcification and hemorrhage from leaking aneurysms. CT is used for major venous structures such as the inferior vena cava, renal, and ileofemoral veins to detect thrombii, invasion by tumor, and congenital abnormalities. Vascular CT scans are usually contrast enhanced and both precontrast and postcontrast scans are obtained.

Nursing Interventions: Client education includes an explanation of the procedure and the need to remain still during imaging. Clients are prepared for the imposing size of the CT scanner and the noninvasive nature of the procedure is emphasized. The ability of the young child to lie still and the need for sedation or restraints is determined. Cardiac CT scanning is not well-suited to infants. If the client is undergoing a contrast-enhanced scan, a history specific as to allergy to iodine or previous reaction to contrast medium is elicited. Clients are frequently NPO 2–4 hours prior to CT scans, especially if contrast medium is to be administered. Clear liquids are sometimes permitted. The client wears a hospital gown, removes all jewelry and prostheses, voids, and goes to the CT room.

Description of the Procedure: This procedure is performed with inpatients and outpatients. The client goes to the CT room. For contrast-enhanced scans, administration of the contrast medium is by IV bolus or infusion drip and may precede scanning by up to 1 hour. The client is supine within the body scanner during the scanning procedure. In order to more clearly identify structures such as the inferior vena cava, the client may be asked to inspire and hold a deep breath or use the valsalva maneuver. This procedure is completed in less than 30 minutes. Results are available after interpretation.

Evaluating Client Response: Postprocedure client and family support is provided. Food and medications are resumed.

LUMBAR SYMPATHETIC BLOCK

This procedure is performed to measure skin response to blocking the sympathetic tracts. A specific consent form is required.

Nursing Diagnoses for clients undergoing lumbar sympathetic block

- Anxiety related to procedure
- Knowledge deficit related to diagnostic process
- Potential alteration in cardiac output related to procedure

Subjective Data: Client complains of pain or intermittent claudication.

Objective Data: Altered physical findings including abnormal pulses, skin color, and temperature.

Assessment: Procaine hydrochloride is inserted into the spinal canal to block the sympathetic rami or sympathetic ganglia. A positive result is achieved when there is resulting vasodilation, i.e., warmer, drier skin, on the extremity on the same side as the injection. A positive result may be used as a basis for further treatment, either medical or surgical. Postprocedure monitoring is required as potential exists for clients to experience shock as blood is suddenly shifted into the peripheral circulation.

Nursing Interventions: Client education includes an explanation of the procedure. The client is prepared for feeling the initial needle insertion as well as tingling or warmth in the legs for several hours following the procedure. Postprocedure monitoring is explained. This procedure is performed in a warm room where the client is kept from being chilled.

Description of the Procedure: This procedure is performed with inpatients and outpatients. The client lies prone or semiprone. The entry site, the second or third lumbar vertebrae, is located and prepared. Local anesthesia may be used to create a wheal. A needle is then inserted into the sympathetic tract and 10–20 ml of 1% procaine hydrochloride is instilled. The client's skin response is measured either by the touch of the tester or by thermocouple, a device that measures skin temperature. This procedure is completed in less than 1 hour. The results are available immediately.

Evaluating Client Response: Following the procedure, the client is monitored for signs of shock. Pulses and blood pressure are assessed every 15 minutes for 1 hour and prn. The client is maintained in a resting position and is kept warm. Postprocedure client and family support is provided.

CONTRAST STUDIES

- **Venography**
- **Digital Subtraction Angiography**
- **Angiography**
- **Coronary Angiography**

Contrast studies are used to determine patency or position of a vessel or chamber in the cardiovascular system. Invasiveness, and, therefore, impact on the client, correlates with the entry and/or infusion site. A specific consent form is required.

Nursing Diagnoses for clients undergoing contrast studies include:

- Alteration in comfort: pain related to procedure
- Anxiety related to procedure
- Knowledge deficit related to diagnostic process
- Potential alteration in tissue perfusion related to procedure
- Potential for injury: allergic reaction related to procedure
- Potential for injury: bleeding related to procedure

Venography (Phlebogram)

Subjective Data: Client complains of pain and swelling.

Objective Data: Altered physical findings including redness, warmth, and swelling in the affected area and a positive Homan's sign.

Assessment: Venography is used to demonstrate nonfilling of a vessel, abnormal valves, traumatic hematoma, as well as its most common use, identifying thrombophlebitis. Phlebography can be used to determine the presence of phlebitis in various sites. Most commonly, the lower extremities need examination; thus, the contrast medium is injected through the dorsal foot vein. For clients with positive phlebograms, treatment will begin immediately.

Nursing Interventions: Client education includes an explanation of the procedure and the importance of remaining still. Clients are told that the injection may be associated with a brief, unpleasant feeling that will pass quickly. A client history specific for previous allergic reaction to contrast media is obtained. Appropriate transportation is provided in order to maintain correct positioning for the suspected affected limb(s). The client wears a hospital gown and removes all jewelry and prostheses.

Description of the Procedure: This procedure is performed with inpatients and outpatients. In the x-ray department, the client is positioned and injected with the contrast medium. The injection may cause a brief painful response. Serial, timed radiographs are obtained. If bilateral films are desired, the procedure is repeated on the opposite side. This procedure is completed in less than 1 hour. Results are available following interpretation.

Evaluating Client Response: If the phlebograms demonstrate phlebitis, medication administration and other therapeutic measures are initiated immediately. Client and family support is provided.

■ Digital Subtraction Angiography (DSA)

Subjective Data: Client complains of pain or shortness of breath.

Objective Data: Altered physical findings, including hypertension and abnormal data from other diagnostic procedures.

Assessment: This procedure uses an image enhancement system, known as mask mode subtraction, to amplify low concentration intravascular iodine signals to obtain data about arterial blood flow. DSA is used to evaluate left ventricular function in clients with ischemic heart disease, suspected coronary artery stenosis, questionable myocardial perfusion and congenital heart disease. Both IV and IA DSA are used. DSA may be performed by itself or in conjunction with other procedures such as coronary angiography.

Nursing Interventions: Client education includes an explanation of the procedure. Client cooperation in lying perfectly still has a major impact on the success of this procedure and this is explained to the client. The need for restraints or sedation in children is determined. A client history specific for allergy to iodine or previous reaction to contrast medium is obtained. For IV DSA, adequacy of kidney function is determined as the client receives 150–250 cc of contrast medium solution over 30–60 minutes. For IA DSA, adequacy of clotting status is determined in order to prevent postprocedure complications. Adjustment in anticoagulant therapy may be needed. Clients may be NPO for 2 hours before the procedure. The client wears a hospital gown, removes all jewelry and prostheses, and voids prior to the procedure.

Description of the Procedure: Both IV and IA DSA are performed with inpatients and outpatients. DSA by intraventricular injection is performed only with inpatients and only in the cardiac catheterization laboratory. Otherwise, the client goes to the radiology department, reclines, and is positioned relative to the fluoroscopic camera. If indicated, the client's ECG is monitored. The mask is recorded and stored by computer. The entry site is prepared. The contrast medium is administered intravenously or intra-arterially. The second image is obtained. Respiratory or other movement may make the mask unsatisfactory. If this occurs, another mask can be obtained after the contrast media has left the region. DSA is completed in less than 1 hour. Results are available following interpretation.

Evaluating Client Response: Following arterial puncture, the client lies supine with the entry site immobilized for 2–4 hours. A pressure dressing or sandbag may be applied to the entry site. The client's blood pressure and pulses, skin color and skin temperature distal to the insertion site are monitored every 15 minutes the first hour, every 30 minutes for the next 2 hours, and every 4 hours thereafter prn. Following both IV and IA DSA, the insertion site is checked for signs of bleeding. Food and medications are resumed and pain medications are administered as needed. Clients are encouraged to increase fluid intake to approximately 2 liters to promote excretion of the contrast medium. Outpatients are instructed to check for postprocedure bleeding and return immediately if any bleeding is noted. Outpatients should not drive home. Client and family support is provided.

■ Angiography (Arteriography, Aortography)

Subjective Data: Client complains of pain, intermittent claudication, numbness, dizziness, or syncope.

Objective Data: Altered physical findings, including altered pulses, bruits, or hypertension, and abnormal data from other diagnostic procedures.

Assessment: Angiography is used in various segments of the arterial system to determine vessel patency or the presence of an aneurysm or collateral circulation. Due to the risk inherent in entering an artery, other procedures precede angiograms in the diagnostic process and attempts are being made to use newer imaging techniques rather than angiography. For arterial pathology, however, angiography remains "the gold standard" and aortograms are considered mandatory before surgery for anuerysmectomy.

Nursing Interventions: Client education includes an explanation of the procedure with emphasis on remaining still. The need for restraints or sedation in children is determined. Clients are told that injection of the contrast media may cause an unpleasant feeling. Clients are told in advance of the routine postprocedure monitoring. A client history specific for previous allergic response to contrast media is obtained. Adequacy of clotting status is determined. Anticoagulant therapy is usually temporarily interrupted. The client is NPO past midnight prior to the procedure and may receive sedation in advance of going to the radiology department. The client wears a hospital gown, removes all jewelry and prostheses, and voids prior to the procedure.

Description of the Procedure: This procedure is performed with inpatients and outpatients when sufficient postprocedure monitoring is available. The client goes to the radiology department. The arterial entry site is located, prepared, and draped. Local anesthesia is administered. The client is instructed not to move until visualization is complete. A catheter is inserted and, via fluoroscopy, is threaded to the intended examination site. Contrast medium is infused via the catheter, and serial, timed radiographs are obtained. Many clients report discomfort during this procedure. The procedure is completed in approximately 1 hour. Interpretation of the results requires detailed viewing of the films.

Evaluating Client Response: Following the procedure, the client is supine with the entry site immobilized for 2–4 hours. A pressure dressing or sandbag may be applied to the entry site. The client's blood pressure and pulses, skin color, and skin temperature distal to the insertion site are monitored every 15 minutes the first hour, every 30 minutes for the next 2 hours, and every 4 hours thereafter prn. The insertion site is checked for signs of bleeding. Food and medications are resumed and pain medications are administered as needed. An increased fluid intake, to approximately 2 liters, is encouraged to promote excretion of the contrast medium. Outpatients should not drive themselves home. Client and family support is provided.

■ Coronary Angiography (Cardiac Catheterization)

Subjective Data: Client complains of chest pain, shortness of breath, or syncope.

Objective Data: Altered physical findings, including rales, edema, hypertension, and abnormal data from other diagnostic procedures, especially exercise testing.

Assessment: This major invasive procedure is used to evaluate cardiac status and to assist in planning future treatment, both medical and surgical. For clients with angina, cardiac catheterization is the definitive method for locating blockages in the coronary artery system. Ventricular wall motion, pressures, and ejection fractions are measured at various points in the cardiac cycle. In addition, response of the heart to stimuli such as medications or external pacing can be measured. Cardiac catheterization is performed before surgical correction of valvular dysfunction. Individual valve function is examined and necessary data concerning ventricular contractility and patency of the coronary arteries are gathered for use during the intraoperative period. Due to the essential nature of the procedure for many clients, prior allergy to contrast media does not necessarily contraindicate the procedure, but will require additional precautions and medications.

Nursing Interventions: Client and family preparation includes an explanation of the procedure. Infants and children too young to cooperate are restrained during the procedure; premedication is frequently used. Clients are told that they will be awake during the procedure and will either be held securely on the catheterization table and be tilted, or will have the camera move around them. Clients are prepared to participate as directed during the procedure. Nurses from the catheterization laboratory can be an effective addition to client and family preparation. Clients and family are told about postprocedure monitoring so they do not misinterpret the routine frequent care. A client history specific to allergy to contrast media is obtained. The client is NPO before the procedure, overnight if the test is scheduled for morning, or after a clear liquid breakfast when an afternoon time is scheduled. Infants who still require feedings every 3–4 hours are kept NPO for only 4 hours prior to the procedure. The client is premedicated with a tranquilizer. Support is provided to reduce client and family anxiety as the test itself is a major procedure and because of its importance in determining further treatment. Family should be encouraged to go to the cafeteria, lounge, etc. and reassured that they will be contacted as soon as the client returns to the room.

Description of the Procedure: Cardiac catheterization is performed with inpatients, and on outpatients in facilities that can provide preprocedure client preparation and posttest monitoring. In the catheterization laboratory, the client is transferred to a cradle-like table and strapped in. If not already in place, a peripheral intravenous line is inserted and the entry site for catheterization prepared. ECG leads are attached to the client. The entry site is shaved, prepared, and draped. The fluoroscope is positioned directly over the client. Using fluoroscopy, a catheter is threaded through the venous system for right-sided catheterization. Also using fluoroscopy, a catheter is threaded through an arterial puncture site for left-sided catheterization and coronary angiography. Once the catheter has been inserted, the entry site is immobilized to prevent untoward catheter movement and/or damage to the blood vessel. If the entry site is the groin, the primary choice, the client may not be too uncomfortable during the procedure. With the arm as insertion site, however, the client may complain of stiffness as the arm is immobilized during the procedure. Contrast media is inserted via the catheter. Catheter movement and gravity may be used to distribute the contrast media to a specific area. Some catheterization tables tilt and the client may experience a falling sensation as the table is tilted although securely restrained to the table. Cardiac catheterization may include manipulating cardiac function by administering medications via external pacing. These cardiac challenges may provoke unpleasant sensations such as hot flashes, cold sensations, nausea, palpitations, and/or feeling one's heart "race." The client may be asked to cough in order to effect vagal response and intrathoracic pressure changes. The time required for this procedure depends on how many aspects of cardiac structure and function are being examined. If access through the blood vessels is difficult, the procedure may take additional time. Cardiac catheterizations may require from 30 minutes to 2 or 3 hours. The cardiologist may give the client and family a brief summary soon after the procedure, but complete results require analysis of the films and may take several hours.

Evaluating Client Response: Vital signs and pulses, skin color, and skin temperature distal to the insertion site are monitored every 15 minutes the first hour, every 30 minutes for 2 hours, every hour for the next 4 hours, and every 4 hours thereafter prn. The puncture site is checked for signs of bleeding. A pressure dressing or sandbag may be applied to arterial puncture sites. The client stays fairly horizontal; movement of the insertion site is prohibited. Food and medications are resumed. The client is encouraged to increase fluid intake to 2 liters in the first few hours to aid in eliminating the contrast media. If the peripheral IV line is intact, it requires monitoring. Outpatients should not drive themselves home. Client and family support in waiting for and dealing with the procedure results is essential.

RENIN STUDIES

Renin studies involve obtaining a blood sample from the inferior vena cava and simultaneous renal vein blood sampling. Aortography is frequently included. A specific consent form is required.

Nursing Diagnoses for clients undergoing renin studies include:

- Anxiety related to procedure
- Knowledge deficit related to diagnostic process
- Potential for injury: allergic reaction related to procedure
- Potential alteration in tissue perfusion related to procedure

Subjective Data: Client complains of headache, fatigue, or throbbing.

Objective Data: Clients with hypertension as described in this section, an abdominal bruit, or equivocal results from ultrasound.

Assessment: Renin studies are performed to determine if renovascular disease is the cause of hypertension. Clients most likely to benefit from this study are under 30, females 35–40 with recent onset, older with deteriorating renal function, or poorly controlled by medication. Renin studies are also indicated for clients who respond positively to treatment with captopril. Renin studies are considered positive if the renin level from one kidney is 1.5 or more times greater than the renin level from the opposite kidney and/or vena cava. Renin studies frequently include aortography to rule out a stenotic lesion in the renal arteries even in the presence of normal renin levels.

Nursing Interventions: Client education includes an explanation of the procedure. The need for sedation or general anesthesia in children is determined. If possible, all other hypertensive and diuretic medications are stopped 2 weeks prior to the procedure. For 3 days before the study, the client eats a 0.5–1.0 g sodium diet and receives diuretic therapy, i.e., diuril 500 mg or hydrodiuril 500 mg twice daily. If the renin study includes aortography, clients are told that injection of the contrast media may cause an unpleasant feeling. A client history specific for previous allergic response to contrast media is obtained. The client is NPO past midnight prior to the procedure. The client wears a hospital gown, removes all jewelry and prostheses, and voids prior to the procedure.

Description of the Procedure: This procedure is performed with inpatients and outpatients. The client arrives early so as to lie supine for 1 hour before the procedure begins. The entry site is located and prepared. The client is instructed not to move until the procedure is complete. Catheters are inserted and, via fluoroscopy, threaded to the inferior vena cava and each of the renal veins. Blood samples are obtained from the renal veins simultaneously and from the vena cava. Frequently, several samplings are performed. Aortography may also be performed. Renin studies are completed in 30–60 minutes. The results are available upon interpretation.

Evaluating Client Response: Following the procedure, the client is supine for 4–6 hours. If arterial puncture has been performed, the entry site is immobilized and a pressure dressing or sandbag may be applied. The client's blood pressure and pulses, skin color, and skin temperature distal to the insertion site are monitored every 15 minutes the first hour, every 30 minutes for the next 2 hours, and every 4 hours thereafter prn. The insertion site is checked for signs of bleeding. Food and medications are resumed and pain medications are administered as needed. An increased fluid intake, to approximately 2 liters, is encouraged to promote excretion of the contrast medium. Outpatients are told to expect minor oozing or pain but to report frank bleeding immediately. Outpatients should not drive themselves home. Client and family support is provided.

3

Clients with Potential for Injury or Infection

The potential for injury or infection can result from many different causes. It may be the primary pathology, be secondary to other pathology, or the result of exposure to some external agent or trauma. A wide range of pathophysiologic, infective or environmental factors may be responsible for triggering an adverse client response. Blood cells, blood forming organs, the reticuloendothelial system and lymphatic network are examined during the diagnostic process. Clients with potential for injury or infection frequently undergo diagnostic testing repeatedly and over a long period of time. Nursing diagnoses for clients during the diagnostic process include psychosocial needs as well as pathophysiologic concerns.

For clients with potential for injury or infection, physical assessment involves several components. A thorough personal history, family history, and history of the present illness are mandatory as is a detailed recording of the client's subjective complaints. The client is questioned regarding all drugs used and exposure to other persons with illness. Detailed questions regarding symptomatology are asked as the onset of illness may be insidious.

Physical examination includes assessing the lymphatic system for enlarged or tender nodes. A positive examination is an indication for further systematic testing and examination of the area being drained. The skin is carefully inspected for signs of overt or subcutaneous bleeding.

LABORATORY TESTS

Laboratory tests are the principal diagnostic tool for clients with potential for injury or infection. Client education is essential since many tests require specific timing, preparation, or other client involvement in order to obtain accurate results. Client support is essential due to the repetitive nature of these tests.

Nursing Diagnoses for clients undergoing laboratory tests include:

- Anxiety related to procedure
- Knowledge deficit related to the diagnostic process

LABORATORY TESTS

Test	Purpose	Normal Values	Nursing Actions
Bleeding time	Assess status re: thrombocytopenia, platelet aggregation, leukemia, aplastic anemia, hemophilia	Adult or child: 1–6 min, Ivy—forearm; 1–3 min, Duke—earlobe; Newborn: 1–5 min, Ivy	Apply direct pressure until bleeding stops
Blood typing	Determine blood type	A, B, AB, O; Rh: + or −	
Cross-matching	Determine compatibility for transfusion	No clumping or hemolysis	May be affected if client previously received incompatible blood type
Coagulation factor concentration test	Assess clotting status		Client should not take aspirin 1 wk prior to test
Factor I Fibrinogen		60–100 mg/ml	
Factor II Prothrombin		10–15% concentration	

Test	Purpose	Normal Values	Nursing Actions
Factor V Proaccelerin		5–10% concentration	
Factor VII Proconvertin		5–20% concentration	
Factor VIII Antihemophilic globulin		30–35% concentration	
Factor IX Thromboplastin		30% concentration	
Factor X Stuart-Power		8–10% concentration	
Factor XI Morphilic		20–30% concentration	
Factor XII Hagemen		0%	
Factor XIII Fibrinstabilizing		1% concentration	
Coagulation time (Lee-White, clotting time)	Assess coagulation, monitor heparin therapy	Adult and child: 5–15 min	Assess for poential bleeding. Pressure may be needed on puncture site for 5 min
Coomb's test (direct or DAGT, indirect or IAGT)	Assess hemolytic disorders ortic screening for transfusion	Negative	Client history is important as many substances can cause a false result
Complement total	Assess inflammatory disease	90–94%	
Complete blood count (CBC)	Assess clotting status, response to infection and inflammation (See appropriate section in Ch. 2 for RBC, HCT, CBC, and RBC indices.)		

(Continued)

LABORATORY TESTS (cont.)

Test	Purpose	Normal Values	Nursing Actions
Platelets	Assess bone marrow, clotting status	Adult: 150,000–450,000/cu mm Child: same as adult Newborn: 150,000/cu mm	
White blood cell count (leukocyte count, WBC)	Assess number and percentage of infection, inflammation and healing	Adult: 4000–11,000/cu mm Child after age 2: same as adult: Newborn: 9000–35,000/cu mm	Do not draw from the same extremity as IV infusion Client history is important as many factors may affect results
Differential			
Neutrophils (polymorphonuclears, polys or segmentals, segs)	Determine presence of infection, inflammation and stress	Older adult: 43–79% Adult: 42–66% or 3000–7000 Child: 50% Infant: 61%	
Band cells (stabs)	Assess presence of recent infection, etc	3%	
Basophils	Assess status as to: polycythemia vera, leukemias, Hodgkin's disease, allergic reactions and stress	0.4–1.0% or 40–100/cu mm	
Eosinophils	Assess reponse to ACTH,	Older adult: 0–0.3% Adult: 1–3% or	

Test	Purpose	Normal Values	Nursing Actions
Eosinophils (cont.)	epinephrine or status as to: allergy, parasitic diseases, leukemia, Hodgkin's disease and eczema	50–400/cc mm Child: 2–3% Newborn: 2–3%	
Lymphocytes	Assess status as to infection, especially viral, and stress	Older adult: 11–48% Adult: 25–33% or 1000–4000/cc mm Child: 30% Newborn: 31%	
Monocytes	Assess status as to bacterial phagocytosis and healing	Older adult: 1–5% Adult: 0–9% or 100–600/cc mm Child: 5–8% Newborn: 6–12%	
Blood culture	Determine presence of pathogens	Negative	Usually drawn serially from different sites to coincide with temperature elevation; must be taken to lab immediately
Erythrocyte sedimentation rate (ESR)	Assess nonspecific inflammation and tissue injury	Women: 0–20 mm/hr Men: 0–15 mm/hr Children: 0–10 mm/hr	
C-reactive protein (CRP)	Assess significance of inflammation and tissue necrosis	Trace	
Fibrin split products (FSP) and	Assess degree of coagulation	< 4.0 μg/ml	

(Continued)

LABORATORY TESTS (cont.)

Test	Purpose	Normal Values	Nursing Actions
fibrin degradation products (FDP)	disorders		
Fibrinogen	Assess ability to form clots; status as to leukemia, liver damage, DIC	Older adult: 470–485 mg/100 ml Adult: 160–300 mg/100 ml Child: 200–400 mg/100 ml Newborn: 150–300 mg/100 ml	
Fibrinopeptide A (FPA)	Assess DIC, leukemia	0.6–1.9 mg/ml	
Human immunodeficiency virus (HIV)	Determine presence of antibodies, indicating prior exposure to virus; positive result is not a diagnosis of AIDS	Negative	
Immunoglobulins	Assess immune system status		Levels vary with age
IgG		600–1700 mg/100 ml	
IgA		65–650 mg/100 ml	
IgM		50–300 mg/100 ml	
IgE		0–200 IU over age 30	
Leukocyte alkaline phosphatase (LAP)	Assess amount of this enzyme in neutrophils, used	40–100	This is drawn from a peripheral smear

Test	Purpose	Normal Values	Nursing Actions
LAP (cont.)	in diagnosing chronic myelogenous leukemia		
Lysozyme (Muramidase)	Assess leukemias, inflammation, infection	2.8–8 μg/ml	
Mononucleosis tests (Monospot, heterophile antibody titer, fluorescent antibody test)	Determine presence of Epstein–Barr antibodies	Negative titer of 1:56 is suspicious >1:224 is diagnostic	
Platelet adhesion	Assess platelet function	50,000–18,000/ cu mm	Client may not take aspirin for 3 wk prior to test
Platelet aggregation	Assess platelet function	Visible <5 min	Do not refrigerate specimen
Platelet volume	Determine platelet size; assess purpura, DIC, anemias, rheumatic disease	8–10 fl 2.5 μm in diameter	
Prothrombin time (protime PT)	Assess coagulant activity of the "extrinsic" system including: factors V, VII, X, fibrinogen, and prothrombin;	100% or also reported in seconds, approximately 11–15, varies in each lab	Increased by warfarin Assess for potential bleeding; pressure on puncture site for 5 min may be required

(Continued)

LABORATORY TESTS (cont.)

Test	Purpose	Normal Values	Nursing Actions
Protime PT (cont.)	monitor warfarin therapy		
Activated partial thromboplastin time (APPT) or partial thromboplastin time (PTT)	Assess all plasma coagulation factors except VII and XII, i.e., stage II clotting disorders such as hemophilia; monitor heparin therapy	APPT: 30–45 sec PPT: 16–25 sec	Increased by heparin Assess for potential bleeding; pressure on puncture site for 5 min may be required
Rh factor	Assess prior to transfusion	Of population: 85–90% are Rh+ 10–15% are Rh−	
Rubella titer (hemaglutination inhibition, HI, HAI)	Determine immunity	Titer >1:8 indicates immunity	
Thrombin clotting time (thrombin time, TT)	Assess stage III clotting	10–20 sec or within 3 sec of control	
Viral antibody test	Determine presence of viral infection	Negative: 1:8 titer Significant: 1:32 or greater	

Please note, these values are guidelines. Check with the laboratory performing the test for absolute values.

DRUG LEVELS

Drug	Effective Concentrations	Peak Action
Amikacin	Peak: 8–16 μg/ml	30–40 minutes after dose
Amoxicillin	Peak: 4μg/ml	2 hr after po dose
Ampicillin	Oral Peak: 3 μg/ml IM Peak: 7–10 μg/ml	2 hr after dose 1 hr after dose
Carbenicillin	IV Peak: 150 μg/ml	>100 μg/ml is maintained by q 4hr administration
Cefamandole	Peak: 20–36 μg/ml	
Cefazolin	Peak: 64 μg/ml	
Cefoxitin	Peak: 22 μg/ml	
Cephalexin	Peak: 16 μg/ml	
Cephalothin	Peak: 20 μg/ml	
Cephradine	Peak: 10–18 μg/ml	
Chloramphenicol	Peak: 10–13 μg/ml	2–3 hr after dose
Chloroquine	Toxic: >.25 μg/ml	
Clindamycin	Peak: 2–4 μg/ml	1 hr after po dose 3 hr after IM dose for adults 1 hr after IM dose for children
Cloxacillin	Peak: 5–10 μg/ml	1 hr after po dose
Cyclosporine	Therapeutic: 100–400 ng/ml	
Dicloxacillin	Peak: 5–10 μg/ml	1 hr after po dose
Doxycycline	Peak: 3 μg/ml	2 hr after dose
Erythromycin	Peak: 0.3–1.9 μg/ml	2 hr after dose
Floxacillin	Peak: 5–10 μg/ml	1 hr after po dose
Flucytosine	Therapeutic: 35–70 μg/ml Toxic: >100 μg/ml	1–2 hr after dose
Gentamycin	Peak: 4–8 μg/ml	30–90 min after dose
Methacycline	Peak: 2 μg/ml	2–4 hr after dose
Methicillin	Peak: 10–20 μg/ml	30–60 min after IM dose
Methotrexate	Toxic: >10 μg/ml	
Minocycline	Peak: 2–3 μg/ml	2–4 hr after dose
Netilmicin	Peak: 4–8 μg/ml	30–90 min after dose
Oxacillin	Peak: 5–10 μg/ml	1 hr after po dose
Penicillin G	Oral Peak: 0.3 μg/ml IM Peak: 1.5 U/ml	30–60 min after dose

(Continued)

DRUG LEVELS (cont.)

Drug	Effective Concentrations	Peak Action
Tetracycline	Peak: 2–3 μg/ml	2–4 hr after dose
Tobramycin	Peak: 4–8 μg/ml	30–90 min after dose
Vancomycin	Peak: 6–10 μg/ml	1–2 hr after IV dose

Please note, these values are guidelines. Check with the laboratory performing the test for absolute values.

ULTRASONOGRAPHY

For clients with potential for injury or infection, ultrasound may be used to diagnose splenic and lymphatic disorders. No specific consent form is required.

Nursing Diagnoses for clients undergoing ultrasonography include:

- Anxiety related to procedure
- Knowledge deficit related to diagnostic process

Subjective Data: Client complains of tenderness, pain, fatigue, and malaise.

Objective Data: Enlargement of spleen or lymph nodes, fever, night sweats, or abnormal laboratory findings.

Assessment: Ultrasound diagnosis of spleen dysfunction is somewhat limited because the spleen is surrounded by the ribs and obscured ultrasonically by gas in the abdomen. Ultrasound is used to assess focal lesions within the spleen. Although normal lymph nodes are too small to be visualized, related blood vessels can be imaged and diagnostic inferences drawn. Ultrasonography is used for assessing abnormal nodes in areas not well-visualized by lymphography, such as the mesenteric and portal nodes.

Nursing Interventions: Client education includes an explanation of the procedure. Specific instructions regarding remaining still and feeling some pressure during the procedure are provided. The different techniques that contribute to increased imaging quality such as changes in position, a distended bladder for pelvic imaging, or performing the valsalva maneuver for imaging nodes along the inferior vena cava are explained.

Description of the Procedure: This procedure is performed with inpatients and outpatients. For ultrasonography, the client assumes a given position and stays still. Access to the skin is required, thus privacy is assured. Conductive oil or gel is used for optimal contact between the transducer and the chest wall. The transducer is moved across the skin with varying pressure according to the structures that need examination. This procedure takes approximately 30–45 minutes. The results are available following interpretation.

Evaluating Client Response: Postprocedure client and family support is provided.

SCINTIGRAPHY

- **Spleen Scan**
- **Bone Marrow Scan**
- **Gallium Scan**

Several scintigraphic studies are used to assess clients with potential for injury or infection. A specific consent form may be required.

Nursing Diagnoses for clients undergoing scintigraphy include:

- Anxiety related to procedure
- Knowledge deficit related to diagnostic process

Spleen Scan

Subjective Data: Client complains of pain or tenderness.

Objective Data: Evidence of trauma to the splenic area, altered physical examination including cyanosis, pallor, tachypnea, or jaundice, and altered laboratory findings.

Assessment: A spleen scan is used to locate mass, hematoma, laceration, or infarction within the spleen. Splenic rupture or accessory spleens can also be located. Currently, Tc-99m is the most commonly used radioisotope for this procedure. Tc-99m is picked up by the reticuloendothelial system. The liver and spleen are both visualized. Scintigraphy is contraindicated during pregnancy and lactation.

Nursing Interventions: Client education includes an explanation of the procedure. Scheduling considerations include 24–48 hours between different nuclear medicine studies in order to reduce potential cross-interference. This study must be performed before any barium testing. All jewelry is removed.

Description of the Procedure: This procedure is performed with inpatients and outpatients. The client lies supine and receives a single IV injection. The scintilation camera is positioned and scanning completed. This procedure takes approximately 30 minutes. The results are available following interpretation.

Evaluating Client Response: Postprocedure support for client and family in dealing with the results is provided.

■ Bone Marrow Scan

Subjective Data: Client complains of fatigue, weakness, or anorexia.

Objective Data: Altered physical findings include the presence of night sweats, enlarged lymph nodes, liver, or spleen, and altered laboratory findings.

Assessment: A bone marrow scan is used to assess myeloproliferative disorders, acute versus chronic hemolysis and to detect focal defects in the bone marrow. It is also used in the staging process for lymphoma, Hodgkin's disease, and other metastases. Scintigraphy is contraindicated during pregnancy and lactation.

Nursing Interventions: Client education includes an explanation of the procedure. The importance of the time interval between injection and scanning is explained. Scheduling considerations include 24–48 hours between different nuclear medicine studies in order to reduce potential cross-interference. All jewelry is removed.

Description of the Procedure: This procedure is performed with inpatients and outpatients. The client receives a single IV injection. Forty-eight hours later, the client lies supine and imaging takes place. Imaging takes approximately $1\frac{1}{2}$ hours. The results are available following interpretation.

Evaluating Client Response: Postprocedure support for client and family in dealing with the results is provided.

■ Gallium Scan

Subjective Data: Client complains of pain, weakness, fatigue, or anorexia.

Objective Data: Altered physical findings including the presence of night sweats, tachypnea, enlarged lymph nodes, liver, or spleen, and altered data from other diagnostic procedures.

Assessment: Gallium-67 is a radioactive isotope that concentrates in certain primary and metastatic neoplasms. Gallium scans are used to determine the presence and to stage neoplasms, especially those associated with bronchogenic carcinoma, Hodgkin's disease, and lymphoma. Gallium scans can also aid in localizing abscesses or inflammatory processes. Scintigraphy is contraindicated during pregnancy and lactation.

Nursing Interventions: Client education includes an explanation of the procedure and of the repeated imaging. Scheduling considerations include 24–48 hours between different nuclear medicine studies in order to reduce potential cross-interference. Gallium scans must be performed before any barium testing. In order to avoid inaccurate results due to stool uptake of gallium, the client may undergo mild bowel preparation consisting of cathartics and/or enemas for 1–3 days prior to injection. Unless contraindicated, the client receives a Fleets enema 1 hour prior to injection. All jewelry is removed. During the procedure, client support is provided, as the wait for the conclusion of the test and the results may seem very long.

Description of the Procedure: This procedure is performed with inpatients and outpatients. The client receives a single IV injection of Ga-67 in a citrate solution. Scanning takes place 24, 48, and 72 hours after injection. For each scan, the client lies supine and is imaged from head to toe. Each imaging takes approximately 1 hour. The results are available after completion of all imaging and following intepretation.

Evaluating Client Response: Postprocedure support for client and family in dealing with the results is provided.

LYMPHANGIOGRAPHY

Clients with potential for injury or infection may undergo lymphangiography, a contrast study to assess the lymph vessels or draining nodes. A specific consent is required.

Nursing Diagnoses for clients undergoing lymphangiography include:

- Alteration in comfort related to diagnostic procedure
- Anxiety related to procedure
- Knowledge deficit related to diagnostic procedure
- Potential for injury: allergic reaction related to procedure
- Potential for injury: complications related to oil embolism

Subjective Data: Client complains of fatigue, weakness, or anorexia.

Objective Data: Abnormal physical examination including enlarged lymph nodes, liver, or spleen, unexplained fever, or night sweats.

Assessment: Lymphangiography consists of slow injection of oily contrast medium containing iodine, followed by radiographs. This procedure is performed for staging purposes in clients with lymphoma or to detect metastases. Lymphangiography is contraindicated in clients with local sepsis or prior removal of draining nodes, since removal causes development of local lymphaticovenous communication and can, therefore, lead to oil embolism. In addition, clients with impaired respiratory function are not candidates for this procedure, since oil emboli to the lungs may occur.

Nursing Interventions: Client education includes an explanation of the procedure and postprocedure monitoring. The need for restraints or sedation of children is determined. Specific instructions are provided regarding the importance of remaining still during the procedure, the use of contrast medium, and the small surgical incision. A client history specific to allergy to iodine is obtained. Sedation may be administered prior to the procedure. If so, appropriate safety precautions are implemented. Fluid restriction may occur prior to lymphangiography so that the client does not need to void while it is in progress. The client removes all jewelry, prostheses, etc., wears a hospital gown, and voids prior to the procedure.

Description of the Procedure: This procedure is performed with inpatients and outpatients. In the x-ray room, the client is positioned according to the area to be examined. Evans Blue Dye is injected intradermally between the first and second digits of the hands or feet. An incision is made 20 minutes later proximally into the skin, and a lymphatic vessel identified. A needle is inserted into the lymphatic vessel and radiopaque oily contrast medium slowly injected. Serial, timed radiographs are obtained as the medium leaves the node. This procedure may take up to 6 hours. Repeat radiographs may be obtained in 24 hours and the lymph nodes will continue to visualize for 4–6 months. The results are available following interpretation.

Evaluating Client Response: Postprocedure evaluation centers on monitoring the client for respiratory distress, chemical pneumonia, neurologic disturbance, or coma. Client assessment, including vital signs and neurologic assessments are performed every 15 minutes the first hour, every 30 minutes for the next 2 hours, and every hour thereafter until stable. Changes in status are reported immediately. Oil emboli do resolve and mortality is rare, but appropriate supportive care is provided while functional impairment exists. Client and family support is provided. Outpatients should not drive themselves home.

BONE MARROW BIOPSY, BONE MARROW ASPIRATION

For clients with potential for injury or infection, bone marrow biopsy may be required to establish a definitive diagnosis. A specific consent form is required.

Nursing Diagnoses for clients undergoing bone marrow biopsy include:

- Alteration in comfort related to procedure
- Anxiety related to procedure
- Knowledge deficit related to diagnostic process

Subjective Data: Client symptomatology will vary with the blood cells affected and may be either somewhat localized or systemic.

Objective Data: Altered laboratory findings on CBC and other diagnostic testing.

Assessment: In bone marrow aspiration, a portion of the bone marrow is removed and analyzed under a microscope. Bone marrow aspiration is performed on clients with clinical evidence of hematopoietic malfunctions including leukemia, anemia, multiple myeloma, Hodgkin's disease or polycythemia. Aspirated bone marrow is examined for cellular activity and for presence or absence of mature and immature cells and precursor cells. Blood cells are examined for normality. Bone marrow is also used to diagnose bacterial or parasitic infections and to monitor therapeutic regimens. Site selection is affected by age. The iliac crest is preferred for adults and children past infancy. Sternal aspiration is not recommended before adolescence. Tibial aspiration is used for infants under 1 year.

Normal values:

M:E ratio (myeloid:erythroid, i.e., granulocytes:total normoblasts):
Adult:4:1; 1–20 years 2.95:1; 1–20 months 5.5:1, birth 1.85:1

Lymphocytes:	Adults 2.7–24%	Children 3–17%
Plasma cells:	Adults 0.1–1.5%	Children 0–2%
Reticulum cells:	Adults 0.1–2%	Children 0.2–2%

Nursing Interventions: Client education includes an explanation of the procedure and the importance of remaining still and resting afterward. Clients are made aware that discomfort may be present during the actual aspiration, but that it subsides when the aspiration process is complete.

Clients may be NPO prior to the procedure. The client may be premedicated with a narcotic such as meperidine or with a minor tranquilizer. Pediatric clients are held securely during this procedure. If the nurse is present during the procedure, client support and technical assistance are provided.

Description of the Procedure: This procedure is performed with inpatients and outpatients. Privacy is assured. The client is positioned according to aspiration site, most commonly the iliac crest or the sternum. The entry site is prepared and local anesthetic is administered to the skin, subcutaneous tissues, and periosteum. The needle is introduced via a stylet. When a marrow biopsy is performed, a small incision allows for entry of the larger biopsy needle. Once the outer cortex of the bone has been pierced and the marrow entered, the stylet is removed and a syringe attached. Approximately 0.5 cc of blood and marrow are aspirated. The syringe is withdrawn and a dressing is applied. The procedure takes less than 15 minutes. Results are available following laboratory analysis and interpretation.

Evaluating Client Response: Postprocedure care includes evaluating the insertion site for bleeding and signs of infection. Pressure is applied, often by having the client lie on the entry site. Pain medication is administered as needed. Tenderness may persist for a few days. Client and family support in dealing with the results is provided.

4

Clients with Impaired Gas Exchange

Impaired gas exchange can result from a wide variety of pathophysiologic causes. Disease may result from anatomical malformation, infection, exposure to toxic agents, neoplasm, allergy, or trauma. Clients may be suddenly unable to breathe or chronically out of breath. Some clients may be caught unaware that illness has developed, whereas others may have smoked for decades. The nursing challenge remains the same: helping the client cope with altered levels of oxygen and carbon dioxide. Nursing diagnoses for these clients during the diagnostic process include psychosocial needs as well as pathophysiologic concerns.

For clients with impaired gas exchange, the diagnostic process begins with thorough physical assessment. A personal history, family history, and history of the present illness are obtained, as is a detailed recording of the client's subjective complaints. The physical examination includes locating bony structures, examining respirations in terms of rate and rhythm, and determining the presence of abnormalities in the respiratory cycle.

For clients with impaired gas exchange, coughing is a significant complaint. The client's cough is evaluated in terms of its character, i.e., dry, productive, etc., onset, relationship to the respiratory cycle, and relationship to exercise, position, or eating. Clients who cough are often assessed while coughing and may be asked to initiate coughing during the physical exam.

Sputum production is a common symptom of impaired gas exchange. Assessment includes relating sputum production to other factors such as position or cough. Several types of sputum analysis are performed in the laboratory. The nurse is responsible for obtaining the correct containers and educating the client as to its use. Specific sputum tests are included in the laboratory tests section.

LABORATORY TESTS

- **Blood Testing**
- **Sputum Testing**

Impaired gas exchange can occur as the primary client problem, or it can be a result of other disease states. Some clients with impaired gas exchange are acutely ill, others will require health care for many years. For all clients, however, teaching is essential because laboratory tests require proper specimens for analysis.

Nursing Diagnoses for clients undergoing laboratory tests include:

- Anxiety related to procedure
- Knowledge deficit related to diagnostic process

LABORATORY TESTS

Test	Purpose	Normal Values	Nursing Actions
Alpha-1-antitrypsin Serum	Assess inflammation, infection, emphysema, liver disease	159–400 mg/100 ml	Clients with elevated cholesterol or triglyceride levels are NPO past midnight prior to this test
Arterial blood gases (ABGs)	Assess respiratory status, acid-base balance	pH: 7.35–7.45 Po_2: 85–100 mm Hg Pco_2: 35–45 mm Hg HCO_3: 18–25 mEq/L Base excess: +2 to −2	Mark lab slip as to any oxygen therapy client received as sample was drawn; place specimen on ice and send to lab immediately; apply pressure to puncture site for 5 min.

(Continued)

LABORATORY TESTS (cont.)

Test	Purpose	Normal Values	Nursing Actions
Carbon dioxide (CO_2) Serum	Determine content, assess acid–base balance	22–34 mEq/L	
Cold agglutinins Serum	Determine level of antibodies, assess stage of illness	Less than 1:32	Specimen is kept at body temperature and taken immediately for analysis
Radio-immuno-assay allergosorbent test (RAST) Serum	Measures amount of specific IgE antibodies	0/1 baseline negative 1–6 indicates positive allergic response	
Serum angiotensin converting enzyme (SACE) Serum	Assess sarcoidosis	23–57 U/ml	Not an accurate tool for persons < 20-yr old.

Please note, these values are guidelines. Check with the laboratory performing the test for absolute values.

DRUG LEVELS

Drug	Effective Concentrations
Ethambutol	Toxic: > 10μg/ml
Terbutaline	Therapeutic: 3 ng/ml
Theophylline	Therapeutic: 10–20 μg/ml

Please note, these values are guidelines. Check with the laboratory performing the test for absolute values.

SPUTUM TESTING

Nursing actions include explanation of the procedure to the client and specific instructions that nasopharyngeal secretions, saliva, or spit are not suitable samples.

The client is given a leakproof screw-capped jar. Some tests require sterile collection containers. The nurse may also apply the mist mask, perform postural drainage, or aspirate a specimen as necessary. Specimens are transported to the laboratory promptly. The rate of pathogen isolation is reduced after only 2–5 hours at room temperature.

Test	Pathogen	Comments
Acid-fast bacilli stain (AFB)	*Mycobacterium tuberculosis*	May be done serially, i.e., three daily first AM samples, done on any fluid or exudate, most commonly sputum or cerebrospinal fluid; requires sterile collection technique
Sputum culture	Normal flora	Requires sterile collection technique
Cytology	Cancer cells	
Gram stain	Various microbes, including: *Streptococcus pneumoniae* *Haemophilus influenzae*	Requires sterile collection technique
Potassium hydroxide wet mount preparation	Blastomycosis, Cryptococcosis, Coccidiomycosis	
Throat culture	Negative: normal flora	Explain and perform procedure; children may need assistance keeping hands away

SKIN TESTING

- **Infectious Agents**
- **Allergens**

When a client with impaired gas exchange has a history suggestive of certain infectious diseases or hyperreactive allergic states, the diagnosis may be supported by a positive response to antigens or allergens placed in the skin, i.e., skin testing. No specific consent form is required.

Nursing Diagnoses for clients undergoing skin testing include:

- Alteration in comfort related to procedure
- Alteration in skin integrity related to procedure
- Anxiety related to procedure
- Knowledge deficit related to diagnostic process

Infectious Agents

Subjective Data: History of exposure to one of the diseases listed in this section; the client complains of fatigue or flu-like symptoms.

Objective Data: Altered physical findings including cough, shortness of breath, weight loss, night sweats, skin lesions, and altered chest x-rays.

Assessment: Skin tests are performed when client history and physical examination are suggestive of an infectious process caused by one of the organisms in the table below. A positive skin test indicates that the client has previously been exposed to the organism and developed an antibody response. Prior multiple skin testing by itself may induce a positive response.

Nursing Interventions: Client education includes an explanation of the procedure. If being done on an outpatient basis, clients are either taught the importance of returning to have the results read or are taught to read the results and notify the appropriate health personnel. All family members are skin tested when any family member is treated for tuberculosis. Nurses are involved in tuberculosis screening for high-risk populations, and they frequently administer skin tests.

Description of the Procedure: Skin testing is done with inpatients and outpatients. The allergen is either scratched or pricked into the skin or injected intradermally. The latter usually results in a larger wheal. The usual site of choice is an area of the forearm that is free from superficial skin disease, hematoma, or other marks that could interfere with accurate interpretation. Each skin test requires less than 1 minute for administration.

Evaluating Client Response: The following chart lists the guidelines for interpreting the results of these tests. Postprocedure nursing responsibilities include test result interpretation and referring clients for treatment as indicated. Client and family support and teaching are provided if the test proves positive.

SKIN TESTS

Name of Test	Organism	Guidelines
Blastomycosis (Gilchrist's disease)	*Blastomyces*	Intradermal injection; site is read in 48–72 hr; negative: no swelling, redness < 5 mm
Brucellosis (Indulant fever)	*Brucella melitensis, abortus,* and *suis*	Intradermal injection; site is read in 48 hr; negative: no redness or swelling
Coccidiodomycosis	*Coccidioides immitises*	Intradermal injection; site is read in 24–72 hr; negative: no swelling, redness < 5 mm
Dick (Scarlet fever)	*Streptococcus pyogenes*	Intradermal injection; site is read in 18–24 hr negative: no more than a pink streak
Frei (Lymphogranuloma venerum)	*Chlamydia*	2 intradermal injections, antigen and control; site is read in 48–72 hr; negative: no redness or swelling; delayed reactions are frequent
Histoplasmosis	*Histoplasma capsulatum*	Intradermal injection; site is read in 24–48 hr; negative: no swelling, redness < 5 mm
Hydatid (Echinococcosis)	*Echinococcus*	Intradermal injection; site is read in 15–20 min; negative: no swelling or redness

(Continued)

SKIN TESTS (cont.)

Name of Test	Organism	Guidelines
Mumps	*Myxovirus*	2 intradermal injections, antigen, and control; site is read in 48–72 hr negative: no redness or swelling
Soft Chancre	*Haemophilus ducreyi*	Intradermal injection; site is read in 72 hr; negative: erythema < 14 mm, swelling < 8 mm; positive reaction may persist for weeks
Toxicoplasmosis	*Toxicoplasma gondii*	2 intradermal injections, antigen and control; site is read in 24–48 hr; negative: swelling or redness < 10 mm
Trichinosis	*Trichinella spiralis*	2 intradermal injections, antigen a control; site is read in 15–20 min; negative: no swelling or redness
Heaf gun	*Myocobacterium tuberculosis*	Injects six punctures simultaneously; site is read in 3–7 days; negative: < 3 papules
Mantoux		Intradermal injection must produce wheal; site is read in 48–72 hr; negative: induration < 5 mm
Tine		Four tines are pressed into skin; site is read in 48–72 hr; negative: no papules
Shick	*Cornybacterium diptheriae*	Intradermal injection; site is read in 48–72 hr; negative: no redness or swelling
Tularemia	*Pasturella tularensis*	Intradermal injection; site is read in 48–72 hr; negative: no redness or swelling

■ Allergens

Subjective Data: Client complains repeatedly of discomfort.

Objective Data: Altered physical findings including coughing, wheezing, sneezing, runny eyes, gastrointestinal, or skin disturbance.

Assessment: Skin testing to determine allergen response is used with clients with a history of repeated symptomatology. Those allergens that provoke hyperreactive response can be identified. Weak skin responses are provoked by scratching the allergen into the skin, whereas stronger, more diagnostic responses are obtained via intradermal injections. These may be performed alone or as parts of a two-phase work-up.

Nursing Interventions: Client education includes an explanation of the procedure. This testing may be uncomfortable for the client; thus, reassurance is provided. All antihistamines and decongestants are withheld for 72 hours prior to testing. This requires detailed discussion with the client and family, as these restrictions encompass a wide range of available medications. The parent is prepared to help the child cope during this uncomfortable procedure. Reassurance, distracting measures, and other support are provided for the child during and after the procedure. Emergency treatment for anaphalactic response is available. Nurses frequently administer these tests.

Description of the Procedure: Each allergen (50 or more may be used at one testing session) is either scratched onto the client's skin or injected intradermally in an orderly manner. The client is then observed for approximately 30 minutes to determine skin response. This procedure takes approximately 45–60 minutes, but depends on the number of allergens involved. The results are available immediately.

Evaluating Client Response: The client is monitored for any difficulty in breathing. Both test administration and the itching associated with the evaluation period make the client quite uncomfortable. Distraction and positive reinforcement as to how well the client is doing may help the client cope. Medications are resumed immediately after the test is complete.

PULMONARY FUNCTION TESTS (PFTs, VENTILATORY FUNCTION TESTS, DIFFUSION TESTS, BRONCHIAL PROVOCATION TESTS)

Pulmonary function tests quantify air movement during respiration. The resulting volumes and flows are used in several different diagnostic processes. A specific consent form may be required.

Nursing Diagnoses for clients undergoing pulmonary function testing include:

- Activity intolerance: fatigue related to procedure
- Anxiety related to procedure
- Knowledge deficit related to diagnostic process

Subjective Data: Client complains of difficulty breathing or fatigue.

Objective Data: Altered physical findings including dyspnea, wheezing, coughing, or sputum production, and altered laboratory findings.

Assessment: PFTs are used to preoperatively screen clients with known risk factors; diagnose clients with unexplained dyspnea or suspected peripheral airway obstruction; determine the status or prognosis of clients with known lung disease; or to screen clients exposed to industrial or environmental pollutants. PFTs are also part of bronchial provocation and medication response testing. Following the initial PFTs, either antigens, methacholine, or histamine in bronchial provocation testing, or a therapeutic agent for medication response testing, are administered. A short wait may be required, and then the PFTs are repeated.

Nursing Interventions: Client education includes an explanation of the procedure and the importance of breathing as directed. If spirometry is to be used, the client is instructed to breathe through the mouth and is informed that nose clips will be applied for assistance. If a body plethysmograph is to be used, the client is prepared for entering the closed box-like structure and is informed that there is constant communication with the tester. For children, the required breathing, nose clips, and/or body plethysmograph can be made into games or otherwise enhanced to ensure client cooperation. Clients with known lung disease should take any medications they use for emergency breathing problems with them to PFT.

Description of the Procedure: Pulmonary function testing is done with inpatients and outpatients. For pulmonary function testing, the client either breathes as directed into a spirometer attached to a measuring device or enters an airtight chamber, a body plethysmograph, in which the air volume is constantly monitored. A health team member tells the client how to breathe according to the test requirements. The time required for PFTs depends on the tests being done and the client's respiratory capability. Data processing and transmitting equipment allow client testing at one location while the results are interpreted at another. This technology serves homebound clients and those who live a long way from pulmonary specialists. Simple screening takes less than 5 minutes, whereas more extensive testing may take 30 minutes. Results are available after interpretation.

Evaluating Client Response: Clients may be quite tired after PFTs. Adequate rest is provided. Client and family support in dealing with the results is provided.

The chart below describes individual components of pulmonary function testing. The normal values are guidelines only, derived from a nonsmoking, nonoverweight, nonelderly population. The results are interpreted by comparing the client's response to the norm for that specific age, weight, height, and sex. Accuracy of the results depends greatly on client cooperation. Some or all measurements are recorded at one time depending on individual client need.

PULMONARY FUNCTION TESTING

Test	Description	Normal
Expiratory measurement		
Vital capacity (VC)	Maximum volume of air exhaled from the point of maximum inspiration	Adult: 4000–4800 ml Child: 43 in: 1200–1250 ml 55 in: 2200–2400 ml
Forced vital capacity (FVC)	Vital capacity with maximum forced expiration	Adult: 4800 ml
Forced expiratory volume (FEV_1, FEV_2, FEV_3)	Forced expiratory volume, in seconds	Adult: FEV_1: 83% of TVC FEV_2: 93% of TVC FEV_3: 97% of TVC FEV_4: 100% of TVC Child: 43 in: FEV_1: 1100 ml 55 in: FEV_1: 2100 ml

(Continued)

PULMONARY FUNCTION TESTING (cont.)

Test	Description	Normal
Expiratory measurement		
Forced expiratory flow (FEF) 200–1200 or Maximum expiratory flow rate (MEFR)	Mean expiratory flow between 200 ml and 1200 ml of the FVC	Adult: 250–450 L/min
Forced midexpiratory flow (FEF) 25–75% or Maximum midexpiratory flow rate (MMEF)	Mean forced expiratory flow during the middle half of the FVC	Adult: 290 L/minute
Forced endexpiratory flow (FEF) 75–85%	Mean forced expiratory flow during the terminal portion of the FVC	
Maximal voluntary ventiation (MVV)	Volume of air expired in a specific period during repetitive maximal effort	Adult: 170 L/min
Expiratory reserve volume (ERV)	Volume of air that can be exhaled after normal exhalation	Adult: 600 L/min
Peak expiratory flow rate (PFR, PEFR)	Maximal flow attainable during forced expiratory volume	Adult: 60 L/min Child: 43 in: 152 L/min 55 in: 300 L/min
Expiratory force (EF)	Expiratory force generated when client blows into a manometer	Adult: +60 cm H_2O
Inspiratory measurement		
Inspiratory capacity (IV)	Maximum amount that can be inhaled from resting expiratory level	Adult: 3000 ml
Forced Inspiratory volume (FIV)	Maximum amount inhaled following maximum expiration	Adult: 3600 ml
Forced inspiration flow (FIF) FIF 100–1200, or Maximal inspiratory flow rate (MIFR)	Mean inspiratory flow during maximal inspiration	Adult: 300 L/min
Inspiratory force (IF)	Amount of negative force generated on in-	Adult: −25 cm H_2O

IF (cont.)	spiration, as demonstrated with manometer	
Other measurements		
Tidal volume (V_t, TV)	Amount inspired or exhaled during normal breathing	Adult: 500 ml
Minute respiratory volume (V_{min})	Amount inspired or exhaled during 1 min	Adult: 6000–7500 ml
Total lung capacity (TLC)	Total volume of air in lungs at the end of maximum inspiration	Adult: 5500–6000 ml Child: 43 in: 1550–1600 ml 55 in: 2950–3050 ml
Residual volume (RV)	Volume remaining in the lungs at the end of maximum expiration	Adult: 1200–1500 ml Child: 43 in: 380 ml 55 in: 650 ml
Functional residual capacity (FRC)	Volume remaining in the lungs at the end normal expiration	Adult: 2400–3000 ml Child: 43 in: 700 ml 55 in: 1350 ml
Flow volume loop (FVL)	Graphic analysis of forced expiratory volume followed immediately by forced inspiratory volume plotted against volume expired	
Diffusion tests	Rates are based on the difference in concentration of gas in inspired and expired air	
Single breath	The amount of gas, a low concentration of CO, or nitrogen, that can be inhaled, held for 10 sec and exhaled	Carbon monoxide: 25 ml/min/mm Hg
Rebreathing	The blood concentration following rapid rebreathing for 90 sec from bag with low concentration CO	
Steady-state	The blood concentration following normal breathing of low concentration of CO for 1 min	17 ml/min/mm Hg

ULTRASONOGRAPHY

Since air prevents conduction of the ultrasonic beam, ultrasound technology is of limited value for clients with impaired gas exchange. No specific consent form is required.

Nursing Diagnoses for clients undergoing ultrasound include:

- Anxiety related to procedure
- Knowledge deficit related to diagnostic process

Subjective Data: Client complains of difficulty breathing and pain.

Objective Data: Abnormal physical findings or chest x-ray.

Assessment: Ultrasound is used to assess clients with suspected pleural effusion. In addition, ultrasonography may be part of the site-selection process for therapeutic pleural aspiration.

Nursing Interventions: Client education includes an explanation of the procedure. The client is prepared for specific positioning and experiencing some pressure during the procedure. Jewelry is removed. Newborns and children may need assistance achieving and maintaining the required position.

Description of the Procedure: This procedure is performed with inpatients and outpatients. Privacy is assured. The client is positioned according to the area to be examined. Conductive oil or gel is applied for optimal contact. The transducer is moved across the skin. Clients may be asked to change position during the procedure. Chest ultrasound is completed in approximately 15 minutes. The results are available following interpretation.

Evaluating Client Response: Client and family support is provided.

MAGNETIC RESONANCE IMAGING (NUCLEAR MAGNETIC IMAGING, MR, NMR)

Thus far, MR has limited use for clients with impaired gas exchange, partly because movement severely degrades imaging; therefore, the scan time can be very long. A specific consent form may be required.

Nursing Diagnoses for clients undergoing MR include:

- Anxiety related to procedure
- Knowledge deficit related to diagnostic process

Subjective Data: Client complains of difficulty breathing, fatigue, or pain.

Objective Data: Altered physical findings including dyspnea or hemoptysis, and altered laboratory or pulmonary function tests.

Assessment: MR is used to differentiate vascular structure, i.e., aneurysm, from hilar, mediastinal, or parenchymal mass. MR is contraindicated in clients with aneurysm clips anywhere in the body because of the potential for movement of ferromagnetic material with rupture of the aneurysm. Clients with pacemakers do not undergo MR because the pacemaker can be affected by radiofrequency pulses.

Nursing Interventions: Client education includes an explanation of the procedure and the need to remain still during imaging. The ability of the child to cooperate is determined. Sedation and restraints are usually required for infants and young children. Clients are prepared for the imposing size of the MR scanner, and the noninvasive nature of the procedure is emphasized. A client health history specific for insertion of aneurysm clips or pacemaker is obtained. The client changes into a hospital gown and removes all jewelry and prostheses.

Description of the Procedure: This procedure is performed with inpatients and outpatients. In the MR room, the client lies supine within the body scanner. Imaging time depends upon image quality and may take 1 hour or more. Results are available after interpretation.

Evaluating Client Response: Client and family support is provided.

SCINTIGRAPHY

- **Perfusion Scan**
- **Ventilation Scan**
- **Radioactive Gas Perfusion Tests**

Scintigraphic examination is frequently used to assess clients with impaired gas exchange. Because scintigraphic imaging is noninvasive, it is used prior to or in place of pulmonary angiography. A specific consent form may be required.

Nursing Diagnoses for clients undergoing scintigraphy include:

- Anxiety related to procedure
- Knowledge deficit related to diagnostic process

Perfusion Scan (Lung Scan)

Subjective Data: Client complains of pain or shortness of breath.

Objective Data: Altered physical findings, including peripheral vein tenderness, swelling, or redness, sputum production, cough, hemoptysis, or abnormal arterial blood gas analysis.

Assessment: Usually performed in tandem with ventilation scans, perfusion scans are used to examine pulmonary vascular circulation and to locate pulmonary emboli. Perfusion scans are also used in determining the extent of disease and/or establishing a prognosis for clients with COPD or carcinoma of the lung. The contrast medium is albumin, labeled with a radioisotope, such as Tc-99m. The perfusion scan usually follows the ventilation scan. Scintigraphy is contraindicated during pregnancy and lactation.

Nursing Interventions: Client education includes an explanation of the procedure. Scheduling considerations include 24–48 hours between different nuclear medicine studies to reduce potential cross-interference. All jewelry is removed.

Description of the Procedure: This procedure is performed with inpatients and outpatients. The client lies supine, to avoid variation in the distribution of the contrast medium due to gravity, and breathes normally as the single IV injection is administered. The client's head may be elevated later, if needed, but the client's position must be the same for the ventilation and perfusion imaging. Several scanning projections may be taken. A ventilation/perfusion scan takes approximately 45 minutes, but may take longer if additional scans are needed. The results are available following interpretation.

Evaluating Client Response: Support for client and family is provided. If the results are positive, therapeutic treatment is initiated immediately.

■ Ventilation Scan

Subjective Data: Client complains of pain or shortness of breath.

Objective Data: Altered physical findings including peripheral vein tenderness, swelling, or redness, sputum production, cough, hemoptysis, or abnormal arterial blood gas analysis.

Assessment: Ventilation scans are used to determine the presence of pulmonary emboli, assess the airways in COPD, or establish a prognosis for clients with carcinoma of the lung. Inert gases—krypton (Kr) or xenon (Xe)—are inhaled by the client, exhaled, and measured. Kr-81m is used to measure tidal breathing because it has two benefits. It can be given by cannula to a client with a tracheostomy and its half-life is so short (13 seconds) that it can be expired without special collection. Xe-133 and Xe-127 are used to assess small airway abnormality. They can provide data about total lung volume at equilibrium and small airway gas retention during washout. Scintigraphy is contraindicated during pregnancy and lactation.

Nursing Interventions: Client education includes an explanation of the procedure with specific instructions regarding positioning, use of the mask or spirometer, and holding maximum inspirations as requested. Scheduling considerations include 24–48 hours between different nuclear medicine studies to reduce potential cross-interference. All jewelry is removed.

Description of the Procedure: Ventilation scans are performed with inpatients and outpatients. The client assumes the same position as for a perfusion scan. The client inhales the inert gas either through a mask tightly fitted over mouth and nose or via a spirometer with nose clips in place. The client takes a maximal inspiration and holds it. The single breath image, which represents ventilation of the lungs, is obtained. For xenon scans, the client then breathes a room air–xenon mixture for 3–5 minutes. A second image, the Equilibrium image, is obtained. This image is an approximate measurement of pulmonary volume. The client then breathes room air to dilute and wash the xenon from the lungs. The expired xenon is collected, as serial images are obtained over the next 7 minutes. Ventilation/perfusion scans take approximately 45 minutes. The results are available following interpretation.

Evaluating Client Response: Support for the client and family is provided. If the results are positive, therapeutic treatment is initiated immediately.

■ Radioactive Gas Perfusion Tests (Radioactive Gas Function Tests)

Subjective Data: Client complains of difficulty breathing.

Objective Data: Altered physical findings including shortness of breath, sputum production, or cough, and abnormal data from other testing including arterial blood gas analysis.

Assessment: These tests are performed to assess regional pulmonary blood flow or function. Inert Xe-133 is either injected intravenously or inhaled. Radiation counters measure the mix of xenon with alveolar air. Uneven distribution in the lungs indicates regional variation in lung perfusion and/or ventilation. Scintigraphy is contraindicated during pregnancy and lactation.

Nursing Interventions: Client education includes an explanation of the procedure with specific instructions regarding injection or inhalation of the radioisotope, and movement of the radiation counter over the client's body. Scheduling considerations include 24–48 hours between different nuclear medicine studies in order to reduce potential cross-interference. All jewelry is removed.

Description of the Procedure: These procedures are performed with inpatients and outpatients. The client either receives a single IV injection containing the radioactive tracer, Xe-133, or inhales a measured amount. Radiation counters then record distribution within the lung. These procedures are completed in less than 15 minutes. The results are available following interpretation.

Evaluating Client Response: Support for client and family is provided.

RADIOLOGY

- **Sinus X-rays**
- **Chest X-rays**
- **Tomograms**

X-rays are valuable tools for assessing clients with impaired gas exchange. The radiographic density of air allows it to be well-visualized and analyzed in relation to surrounding bone, soft tissue, and fat. A specific consent form may be required.

Nursing Diagnoses for clients undergoing radiography include:

- Anxiety related to procedure
- Knowledge deficit related to diagnostic process

Sinus X-rays

Subjective Data: Client complains of altered breathing, pain, or fatigue.

Objective Data: Altered physical findings including fever, tenderness to palpation, and nasal discharge.

Assessment: X-rays are used to assess inflammation or blockage within the sinuses. When such pathology exists, normal air distribution in the sinuses is disrupted. A series of radiographs is taken, with different client/camera positions, in order to provide complete examination of the paranasal, maxillary, frontal, sphenoid, and ethnoid sinuses.

Nursing Interventions: Client education includes an explanation of the procedure. Clients are prepared to change position for the many views required. All jewelry, eye glasses, hearing aids, etc. are removed.

Description of the Procedure: This procedure is performed with inpatients and outpatients. The client is positioned relative to the camera. Client position may be changed after each radiograph. The series is completed in less than 15 minutes. The results are available following interpretation.

Evaluating Client Response: Client and family support is provided.

Chest X-Rays (CXR)

Subjective Data: Client complains of altered breathing, pain, or fatigue.

Objective Data: Altered physical findings including cough or hemoptysis and altered pulmonary function testing.

Assessment: Chest x-rays are obtained for screening purposes, as a preoperative baseline and to monitor changes in status. The heart, lungs, mediastinum, pulmonary vessels, trachea, proximal bronchi, pleura, and diaphragm are visualized. Pathologic processes such as calcification, consolidation, cysts, fibrosis, lymphadenopathy, neoplasms, pleural effusion, pneumo/hemothorax, or tuberculosis can be identified. The location of tubes or catheters can be ascertained. Routine chest x-rays include a posteroanterior (PA) and a lateral view. Oblique views are also commonly used. For other diagnostic purposes, other views requiring different client and camera positions may be obtained. The anteroposterior (AP) view is used for clients confined to bed, whereas horizontal views may be used to confirm clinical suspicion of pleural effusion.

Nursing Interventions: Client education includes an explanation of the procedure and the need for different positions. The client wears a hospital gown and removes all jewelry, etc.

Description of the Procedure: This procedure is performed with inpatients and outpatients and may be performed bedside for acutely ill clients. The client is positioned relative to the camera according to the desired view. In order to provide optimal visualization, the client inspires and holds a deep breath. This test takes less than 10 minutes. The results are available following interpretation.

Evaluating Client Response: Client and family support is provided.

■ Tomography (Linear Tomography, Laminagraphy, Planigraphy, Stratigraphy, Body Section Roentgenography)

Subjective Data: The client experiences changes in breathing pattern, difficulty in swallowing, pain, or fatigue.

Objective Data: Altered physical findings include cough or hemoptysis and altered pulmonary function testing.

Assessment: Tomograms are the procedure of choice for assessing nodules or calcifications and for evaluating suspected cavitation in a pulmonary mass or infiltrate. In the mediastinum, tomograms are used to differentiate masses from vessels and to identify displacement of air–soft tissue interfaces. Client/camera position depends on the desired plane.

Nursing Interventions: Client education includes an explanation of the procedure and the need for several film exposures. The client wears a hospital gown and removes all jewelry, etc.

Description of the Procedure: This procedure is performed with inpatients and outpatients. The client is positioned relative to the camera according to the desired view. In order to provide optimal visualization, the client inspires and holds a deep breath. This process is repeated for each exposure. Tomography takes less than 30 minutes. The results are available following interpretation.

Evaluating Client Response: Client and family support is provided.

COMPUTED TOMOGRAPHY (CT, COMPUTERIZED AXIAL TOMOGRAPHY, CAT SCAN, EMI)

Computed tomography is a valuable tool for assessing clients with impaired gas exchange. The nasopharynx and larynx including cartilage and soft tissue can be evaluated. A specific consent form may be required.

Nursing Diagnoses for clients undergoing CT include:

- Anxiety related to procedure
- Knowledge deficit related to diagnostic process
- Potential for injury: allergic reaction related to procedure

Subjective Data: Client complains of difficulty breathing, pain, or fatigue.

Objective Data: Altered physical findings including cough, and abnormal data from chest x-ray or pulmonary function testing.

Assessment: CT is the method of choice for locating small lung masses and for determining if a mass is neoplasm, fatty cyst, calcification, blood, or edema. Recent CT advances allow for distinguishing aortic aneurysm from aortic dissection. Hilar adenopathy can be assessed, as can the mediastinum and the thymus in clients under 40 years. CT can be performed on clients with advanced life support systems and is also used to direct percutaneous biopsy or drainage procedures. CT scans consist of several views. Scatter radiation is limited, however, so that each exposure receives only its own radiation.

Nursing Interventions: Client education includes an explanation of the procedure and the need to remain still during imaging. The ability of children to cooperate by lying still and/or the need for sedation or restraints is determined. If the client is undergoing a contrast-enhanced scan, a history specific to allergy to iodine or previous reaction to contrast medium is elicited. Clients are prepared for the imposing size of the CT scanner and the noninvasive nature of the procedure is emphasized. Clients are frequently NPO 2–4 hours prior to CT, especially if undergoing a contrast-enhanced scan. Clear liquids are sometimes permitted. The client changes into a hospital gown, removes all jewelry and prostheses, voids, and goes to the CT room.

Description of the Procedure: This procedure is performed with inpatients and outpatients. For contrast-enhanced CT scanning, administration of the contrast medium, either by IV bolus or by infusion drip, precedes scanning by up to 1 hour. During scanning, the client is supine within the body scanner. The client is usually asked to inspire slowly and hold a deep breath. Occasionally, the client is asked to perform the valsalva maneuver. Imaging requires less than 5 minutes and the procedure is completed in less than 30 minutes. Results are available after interpretation.

Evaluating Client Response: Medications and food are resumed. Client and family support is provided.

CONTRAST STUDIES

- **Digital Subtraction Angiography**
- **Pulmonary Angiography**
- **Bronchography**

Clients with impaired gas exchange undergo contrast studies only after the results of other diagnostic testing are inconclusive. A specific consent form is required.

Nursing Diagnoses for clients undergoing contrast studies include:

- Alteration in comfort related to procedure
- Anxiety related to procedure
- Knowledge deficit related to diagnostic process
- Potential alteration in perfusion related to procedure
- Potential for injury: allergic reaction related to procedure
- Potential ineffective breathing pattern related to procedure

Digital Subtraction Angiography (DSA)

Subjective Data: Client complains of pain or shortness of breath.

Objective Data: Clinical evidence suspicious for pulmonary embolism, including hemoptysis or peripheral vein involvement, and equivocal results from ventilation/perfusion studies.

Assessment: This procedure uses an image enhancement system, known as "mask mode subtraction," to amplify low concentration intravascular iodine signals to obtain data about arterial blood flow. IV DSA is being used with success as a means of evaluating clients with suspected pulmonary embolus. IV DSA poses less risk than conventional pulmonary angiography. However, a client must be able to suppress his or her cough upon coaching, must not be extremely dyspneic, or have low cardiac output, and must be able to hold his or her breath and lie still for 20 seconds.

Nursing Interventions: Client education includes an explanation of the procedure. The ability of the client to lie perfectly still, hold his or her breath, and not cough has a major impact on the success of this procedure and this is explained to the client. The client is prepared to expect to feel the urge to cough during contrast medium insertion, but to fight this urge and continue holding the breath as directed. Due to the need for absolute immobility, this procedure is not suited for infants and young children. A client history specific for allergy to iodine or previous reaction to contrast medium is obtained. Adequacy of kidney function is determined, via BUN and creatinine, as the client receives 150–250 cc of contrast medium solution over 30–60 minutes. Clients may be NPO for 2 hours before the procedure. Premedication is not usually necessary, although extremely anxious clients may receive IV diazepam. The client wears a hospital gown, removes all jewelry and prostheses and voids prior to the procedure.

Description of the Procedure: IV DSA is performed with inpatients and outpatients. The client goes to the radiology department, reclines, and is positioned relative to the fluoroscopic camera. If indicated, the client's ECG is monitored. The mask is recorded and stored by computer. The entry site is prepared. The contrast medium is administered intravenously or intra-arterially. The second image is obtained. Respiratory or other movement makes the mask unsatisfactory. If this occurs, another mask can be obtained after the contrast medium has left the region. DSA is completed in less than 1 hour. Results are available following interpretation.

Evaluating Client Response. Following IV DSA, the insertion site is checked for signs if bleeding. Food and medication are resumed and pain medications are administered as needed. Clients are encouraged to increase fluid intake to approximately 2 liters to promote excretion of the contrast medium. Outpatients are instructed to check for postprocedure bleeding and return immediately if any bleeding is noted. Outpatients should not drive home. Client and family support is provided.

■ Pulmonary Angiography

Subjective Data: Client complains of pain or shortness of breath.

Objective Data: Demonstrated clinical evidence of pathology, particularly pulmonary embolism, including hemoptysis or peripheral vein involvement, and equivocal results from ventilation/perfusion studies.

Assessment: Pulmonary angiography is performed to obtain a definitive diagnosis when the client risk of treatment or nontreatment is high. It is performed preoperatively on candidates for pulmonary embolectomy or planned interruption of the vena cava, on infants and children with suspected congenital abnormalities of the pulmonary vasculature, or in young, previously normal people facing a lifetime of uncertainty. Balloon-selective pulmonary angiography can be used for selected regional pulmonary angiography.

Nursing Interventions: Client education includes an explanation of the procedure and the need to remain still. The ability of the child to cooperate and/or the need for sedation or restraints is determined. Clients are prepared to feel the contrast medium being inserted and to expect postprocedure monitoring. A history specific for prior allergic reaction to radiopaque dye is obtained. Clients are NPO past midnight prior to the procedure. Clients may receive a sedative prior to pulmonary angiography, and if so, appropriate safety precautions are implemented. The client wears a hospital gown, removes all jewelry and prostheses, and voids prior to the procedure.

Description of the Procedure: This procedure is performed with inpatients and outpatients when sufficient postprocedure monitoring is available. The client goes to the x-ray department and lies supine on the table. The entry site is prepared and draped. Local anesthesia is administered. A catheter is inserted intravenously and threaded via fluoroscopy through the right side of the heart and into the pulmonary artery. Contrast medium is inserted through the catheter and serial timed radiographs obtained. Many clients cough and/or report a warm, flushed feeling associated with contrast medium injection. This procedure is completed in approximately 1 hour. Interpretation of the results requires detailed viewing of the films.

Evaluating Client Response: Following the procedure, the client is monitored for potential adverse complications from catheter insertion, irritation of the myocardium, congestive heart failure, or allergic response to medications. Vital signs are monitored every 15 minutes the first hour, every 30 minutes for the next 2 hours, and every hour for 4 hours, and prn thereafter, with specific attention to cardiac rate and rhythm. The lungs are assessed frequently. The entry site is monitored for bleeding. Medication and food are resumed. Fluid intake is encouraged to promote excretion of the contrast medium. Outpatients should not drive themselves home. Emotional support for client and family is provided.

■ Bronchography

Subjective Data: Client complains of frequent coughing paroxysms, fatigue, or weight loss.

Objective Data: Thick sputum containing pus and a high bacterial count; abnormal physical findings including hemoptysis, rales, rhonchi and sinusitis, and abnormal findings from other diagnostic procedures.

Assessment: Bronchography is used to assess patency and caliber of the bronchial tree in clients with suspected bronchiectasis. As this clinical entity becomes less common, this procedure is performed less frequently.

Nursing Interventions: Client education includes an explanation of the procedure and specific instructions regarding postural drainage. The ability of the child to cooperate is determined. Restraints or general anesthesia may be required. The importance of client cooperation in coughing and deep breathing following the procedure is emphasized. The client is NPO for 6–8 hours prior to the procedure. Sedation and/or atropine are administered prior to the procedure to suppress the cough reflex and to inhibit bronchial secretions. Appropriate safety precautions are implemented. All jewelry and prostheses are removed and the client voids prior to the procedure.

Description of the Procedure: This procedure is performed with inpatients and outpatients. First, vigorous postural drainage is performed to clear the bronchi of secretions. The client gargles with local anesthesia to prevent gagging and to decrease discomfort. A bronchoscope or catheter is introduced into the trachea and the contrast medium, either radiopaque oil or water soluble dye, is instilled. The client is tilted so that the contrast medium runs along the bronchial walls to the desired location. A series of radiographs is obtained. Upon completion, the client immediately receives vigorous postural drainage to clear the airways and promote expectoration of the contrast medium. This procedure is completed in 1 hour. The results are available following interpretation.

Evaluating Client Response: Postprocedure monitoring centers on the potential for aspiration and regurgitation, as well as the importance of removing all contrast medium from the bronchi. Postural drainage is performed immediately following the procedure and periodically thereafter. Large volume nebulizers, coughing, and deep breathing are used to help the client eliminate the contrast medium. The presence of contrast medium in the sputum is documented. The client is monitored for signs of dyspnea or cyanosis and return of the gag reflex. The client remains NPO until this reflex is demonstrated. Oral intake begins with ice chips. Close monitoring is maintained to be certain that the client experiences no difficulty in swallowing. Follow-up films are taken periodically to determine complete removal of all contrast medium. Outpatients should not drive themselves home. Emotional support for the client and family in dealing with the procedure and the results is provided.

DIRECT VISUALIZATION

Bronchoscopy is direct visualization of the tracheobronchial tree. A specific consent form is required.

Nursing Diagnoses for clients undergoing bronchoscopy include:

- Alteration in comfort related to procedure
- Anxiety related to diagnostic process
- Knowledge deficit related to procedure
- Potential for injury: aspiration related to procedure

Subjective Data: Client complains of difficulty breathing, fatigue, or anorexia.

Objective Data: Altered physical findings including cough or hemoptysis and abnormal data from other laboratory and diagnostic tests.

Assessment: Two different bronchoscopes are in use. The rigid bronchoscope was the first developed. The fiberoptic bronchoscope is flexible, smaller, and has better optics. It is tolerated better by clients. Bronchoscopy is an invasive procedure, and as such is performed after other tests have provided insufficient data for a definite diagnosis. Bronchoscopy is used diagnostically to assess strictures or inflammations; examine pooled secretions; perform biopsy via biting forceps, curette or brush method; determine whether a tumor can be surgically resected; or assess bleeding areas. There are also several surgical uses for bronchoscopy including removal of foreign bodies, secretions, or lesions.

Nursing Interventions: Client education includes an explanation of the procedure and of postprocedure monitoring. The ability of the child to cooperate and the need for restraints is determined. Clients are NPO past midnight and usually receive atropine to dry secretions and a sedative or narcotic prior to the procedure. Appropriate safety precautions are implemented. An IV infusion may be started. If bronchoscopy is done at the bedside, the nurse provides client reassurance and technical assistance during the procedure.

Description of the Procedure: This procedure is performed with inpatients and outpatients and may be performed bedside. Bronchoscopy for diagnostic purposes is usually performed under local anesthesia. The client either gargles with lidocaine or it is sprayed on the pharnyx. Lidocaine may also be dropped on the glottis, vocal cords, and into the trachea. Rigid bronchoscopes are inserted through the mouth, whereas fiberoptic bronchoscopes are usually inserted through the nares. Length of time for the procedure depends on what is done during bronchoscopy and ranges from 10 minutes to about 1 hour. The results from visualization are available immediately, although biopsies or other tests requiring laboratory analysis are of longer duration.

Evaluating Client Response: The client is monitored every 15 minutes the first hour, every 30 minutes the next hour, and every hour thereafter until vital signs are stable. Dyspnea, cyanosis, arrhythmias, and/or tachycardia are reported immediately. If an excision was performed, some hemoptysis may be expected, otherwise, this is considered an adverse reaction and the physician is notified. The client is NPO until return of the gag reflex, which is determined by light touch of a tongue blade to the uvula. This may take several hours, depending on the sedation and anesthesia used. Oral intake then begins with ice chips. Close monitoring is maintained to be certain the client swallows with no difficulty. The client may experience postprocedure discomfort and analgesia is administered as needed. If an IV line has been inserted, it requires monitoring. Postprocedure emotional support is provided for client and family.

BIOPSY

- **Transtracheal Aspiration**
- **Pleural Biopsy**

Examination of a biopsy sample represents the definitive diagnostic method for many pathophysiologies. A specific consent form is required.

Nursing Diagnoses for clients undergoing biopsy include:

- Alteration in comfort related to procedure
- Anxiety related to diagnostic process
- Knowledge deficit related to procedure
- Potential for impaired gas exchange related to procedure

Transtrachial Aspiration (TTA)

Subjective Data: Client complains of pain, difficulty breathing, and fatigue.

Objective Data: Abnormal physical findings including fever, sputum production, cough, cyanosis, mild-to-moderate hemoptysis, or abnormal pulmonary function tests.

Assessment: Transtracheal aspiration is used to obtain a sputum specimen from the lower airway when contamination by pathogens in the oral cavity poses a threat to diagnostic accuracy. This procedure is contraindicated for clients with severe hemoptysis, bleeding problems, severe hypoxemia, or those who are unable to cooperate.

Nursing Interventions: Client education includes an explanation of the procedure and the importance of holding still. The ability of the child to cooperate and the need for sedation or restraints is determined. Post-procedure monitoring is discussed. If present during the procedure, the nurse helps the client remain still, offers emotional support, and assists other personnel as needed.

Description of the Procedure: TTA is performed with inpatients and outpatients. Client privacy is assured. The client is placed in a supine position with the neck hyperextended. If the client is receiving oxygen, it is continued during the procedure. The notch between the lower border of the thyroid cartilage and the cricoid cartilage is located and prepared. Local anesthesia is administered. A 14-gauge needle of an intracath is inserted, advanced a few millimeters, and fixed. Attached to either a syringe or by Y-connector to a sputum trap, the catheter is inserted. Aspiration is completed and the intracath withdrawn. Pressure is applied to the puncture site for several minutes. The procedure is completed in less than 15 minutes. The results are available following laboratory analysis.

Evaluating Client Response: Vital signs are monitored every 15 minutes the first hour, every 30 minutes for the next 2 hours, every hour for the next 4 hours and prn. The client's respiratory rate and rhythm are assessed and the puncture site is checked for bleeding. The client is monitored for potential adverse reactions to the puncture, to catheter placement in the lower airway, or for vasovagal reaction. Emotional support is provided for client and family.

■ Pleural Biopsy (Lung Biopsy, Thoracentesis, Needle Aspiration)

Subjective Data: Client complains of pain, difficulty breathing, and fatigue.

Objective Data: Abnormal physical findings including breathing patterns, lung sounds, fever, sputum production, cough, cyanosis, hemoptysis, or abnormal pulmonary function or other testing.

Assessment: Percutaneous lung biopsy, thoracentesis, and pleural biopsy are similar techniques, with similar client preparation, participation, and postprocedure nursing care. Lung biopsy is performed for clients who have radiographic evidence of disease but who refuse thoracotomy until a definite diagnosis is made, for clients in whom a thoracotomy is hazardous due to other disease, or for clients who are under 35 to exclude malignancy in a solitary nodule. Thoracentesis is performed to obtain pleural fluid for analysis. Therapeutic thoracentesis is performed to relieve intrathoracic pressure associated with excess fluid in the lung. Some institutions are exploring inserting a fiberoptic bronchoscope into the pleural space as a biopsy technique. The normal value for pleural fluid is less than 20 ml.

Nursing Interventions: Client education includes an explanation of the procedure and the importance of not moving during the procedure. The ability of the child to cooperate and the need for sedation is determined. The nurse may hold the child in position during the procedure. The postprocedure monitoring and chest x-ray are explained. A preprocedure chest x-ray and baseline vital signs are obtained for postprocedure comparison. If present during the procedure, the nurse helps the client remain still, offers emotional support, and assists other personnel as needed.

Description of the Procedure: Lung or pleural biopsy by needle aspiration can be done with the patient lying still in any position. Client privacy is assured. Client position depends on the area being biopsied. The client may sit upright and lean over a bedside table or may lie on the unaffected side with the bed elevated 30 to 45 degrees. The entry site is located and prepared. Local anesthesia is administered slowly, at first intradermally to create a wheal, and then deeper in the intercostal space to anesthetize the parietal pleura. This syringe is withdrawn and the biopsy needle inserted through the skin wheal. Needle insertion for biopsy may be guided by fluoroscopy. The biopsy sample and/or pleural fluid is aspirated, with suction applied via a stopcock, if needed. The needle is withdrawn. A dressing is applied to the entry site. The procedure is completed in less than 15 minutes. The results are available following laboratory analysis.

Evaluating Client Response: The client's respiratory rate and rhythm, pulse and blood pressure are assessed every 15 minutes the first hour, every 30 minutes for the next 2 hours and prn. The client is observed for bleeding at the entry site and excessive blood in the sputum. The client is monitored for signs of potential shock, pneumothorax, mediastinal shift, or infection. A postprocedure chest x-ray is obtained. Emotional support is provided for client and family.

5

Clients with Alterations in Nutrition, Metabolism, and Elimination

For each client, optimal nutrition depends on many interrelated bodily functions. Intake of nutrients, digestion, absorption, transport, regulatory mechanisms, and excretion of nonmetabolized substances are all essential components of adequate nutritional status. The client's alterations in nutrition, metabolism, and elimination may arise from dysfunction in any one or more areas in the alimentary chain. These clients present complex challenges in diagnosis and nursing care. Alterations in any one function affects the others. Society and culture exert strong influences on the voluntary aspects of nutrition and elimination, whereas a wide variety of pathophysiologic states affect nutrient intake, metabolism, and elimination. Nursing diagnoses during the diagnostic process address psychosocial needs in addition to pathophysiologic concerns.

For clients with alterations in nutrition, metabolism, and elimination, complete assessment involves several components. A thorough personal history, including customary pattern of intake and elimination, family history and history of the present illness is mandatory, as is a detailed recording of the client's subjective complaints. Oral health is included in this process. Physical examination of the abdomen includes inspection, auscultation, percussion, and palpation. Other areas of the body are examined for signs or symptoms of alterations in nutritional status.

For clients with alterations in nutrition, metabolism, and elimination, stool examination is essential. Feces are assessed in terms of amount, color, consistency, frequency, odor, and the presence of blood, mucus, or undigested food. Stool samples may be cultured for microorganisms or parasites. The effects of diet, medication, and/or pathophysiology are considered. Testing for occult blood may be performed anywhere with the proper supplies. Nurses frequently do this analysis and report results immediately. Occult blood testing may be performed as a specific diagnostic test or as a wide-scale screening mechanism for bowel disease, specifically carcinoma. Clients may be given dry paper slides along with instructions for obtaining the sample at home and mailing it for analysis.

LABORATORY TESTS

Clients with altered nutritional status undergo multiple laboratory tests on various body substances. Client education is essential, since many tests require specific timing, preparation, or other client involvement for accurate analysis. Inadequate client knowledge related to these tests can be costly in terms of time, efficiency, and expense.

Nursing Diagnoses for clients undergoing laboratory testing include:

- Anxiety related to procedure
- Knowledge deficit related to diagnostic process
- Potential alteration in comfort related to procedure

LABORATORY TESTS

Test	Purpose	Normal Values	Nursing Actions
Acetoacetate (acetone) Serum	Assess for acidosis, toxemia, altered diet	0.3–2.0 mg/100 ml	
Aldolase Serum	Assess hepatic muscular status, MI, malignancy	171–474 mU/ml	
Alkaline phosphatase (ALP) Serum	Assess bone, status; renal, hepatic, intestinal and biliary tract status	Adult: 30–115 mU/ml Puberty: 30–165 mU/ml Child: 60–300 mU/ml	Assess child for bone growth as values are related to this; client is NPO 8–12 hr prior to test
Ammonia (NH_4) Serum	Assess hepatic and renal function	17–80 μg/100 ml; Varies with lab	Client may be NPO 8 hr prior to test; place specimen on ice as soon as drawn

(Continued)

LABORATORY TESTS (cont.)

Test	Purpose	Normal Values	Nursing Actions
Amylase Serum	Assess pancreatic, renal or salivary gland status	20–110 mU/ml	If abdominal or pleural fluid is used, more client care will be required
Urine		1–17 U/hr	Urine sample may be random, 2 hr, 12 hr, or 24 hr;
Bilirubin (icterus index) Serum	Assess hepatic, biliary tract or hemolytic status	Total: Adult: 0.2–1.2 mg/100 ml Newborn: 1.0–12.0 mg/100 ml Indirect/ Unconjugated: Adult: 0.1–0.8 mg/100 ml Newborn: 1–11 mg/100 ml Direct/Conjugated: Adult: 0.1–0.4 mg/100 ml Newborn: 1.0–12.0 mg/100 ml Icterus index: 4–6 U	Levels affected if drawn within 24 hr of radiopaque dye injection; Specimen is kept out of bright light; refrigerate specimen if not being immediately examined
Urine		Negative	Testing tablets are kept cool and dry; urine sample must be fresh
Calcitonin Serum	Assess malignancy, especially thyroid	50–500 pg/ml	Client is NPO past midnight prior to test
Carcinoembryonic antigen (CEA) Serum	Screening tool for many carcinomas, including colorectal and breast	0–2.5 mg/ml	

Test	Purpose	Normal Values	Nursing Actions
Carotene (vitamin A, retinol) Serum	Assess nutritional status, absorption	50–300 μg/100 ml 63–273 IU/100 ml	
Copper	Assess hepatic function		
Serum		70–165 μg/100 ml	
Urine		20–70 μg/24 hr	
C-peptide Serum	Assess beta cell secretory function	0.9–4.2 mg/ml	Client is NPO 8 hr prior to test
Fecal culture	Determine presence of pathogens	No pathogens, usual organisms only	Refrigerate sample if testing is not done immediately
Fecal fat/mucus/pus	Determine presence		
Qualitative		Fat: 1+, i.e., few fat spheres, smaller than RBCs; Mucus: negative Pus: negative	Refrigerate sample if testing is not done immediately
Quantitative		3–5 g fat/24 hr	Client takes controlled fat (80–100 g/day) diet × 2 days; may take stool softener to promote excretion; Stool collected for 24–72 hr; use weighted resealable container
Folic acid (folate) Serum	Determine level and assess malnutrition, anemia, malabsorption	Adult: >3 ng/ml Indeterminate: 1.5–3 ng/ml Deficient: <1.5 ng/ml	Client is NPO 8 hr prior to test

(Continued)

LABORATORY TESTS (cont.)

Test	Purpose	Normal Values	Nursing Actions
Galactose-1-phosphate uridyl transferase Serum	Assess galactosemia	>18 U activity/g Hemoglobin	
Gastrin Serum	Assess intestinal disease	Fasting: 50–155 50–155 pg/ml Postprandial: 80–170 pg/ml	
Glucose fasting Serum bG chemstrip Capillary whole blood	Assess pancreatic, liver, or endocrine status, diabetes mellitus,	Adult: 65–110 mg/100 ml Child: 60–105 mg/100 ml Newborn: 20–80 mg/100 ml	Client is NPO overnight prior to test being drawn; teach client how to perform test
2-hr postprandial (2-hr PP) Serum	hypoglycemia, malabsorption, Cushing's syndrome; response to glucose/food intake	Glucose level should be within normal limits	Eating and specimen collection schedules must be coordinated
Urine (sugar acetone, AC urine, DU)		0–15 mg/100 ml Negative by color change test	Double voided specimens are more accurate; refrigerate specimen if not tested immediately; teach client how to perform test
24-hr urine		100 mg/100 ml	Keep collection container on ice
Glucagon serum	Assess pancreatic, renal status	50–200 pg-ml	
Growth hormone (hGH, somatotrophin) Serum	Assess pituitary status	Adult Female: 0–15 μg/ml Adult Male: 0–10 μg/ml Child: 0–10 μg/ml	Clients are NPO past midnight prior to test

Test	Purpose	Normal Values	Nursing Actions
Guaiac (fecal or occult blood, hemoccult, hematest) Feces	Determine presence of blood that is not visible	Negative	Teach client to use correct method for package tests
Hemoglobin A1c (glycosylate hemoglobin) Serum	Determine pattern of blood glucose levels over time	4.3–6.7%	
Hepatitis antigen (HAA, HB)	Determine previous infection by hepatitis B virus	Negative	Avoid direct contact with client's blood
Hexsaminidase Total serum	Assess diabetes mellitus, Tay-Sachs disease	333–375 nM/ml/hr	
Hexsaminidase A Serum		49–68% of total	
Indocyanine green Serum	Assess hepatic function	500–800 ml/sq m body surface/min	
Isocitric dehydrogenase Serum	Assess hepatic function	50–180 units	
Ketone bodies (acetone) Serum	Assess metabolic acidosis, diabetes mellitus	Adult and child: 0.3–2 mg/100 ml (acetone) 2–4 mg/100 ml (ketone) Newborn–1 wk: slightly higher	Use uncontaminated fresh specimen
Urine		Negative, no color change	Teach client how to perform this test
Lactic acid dehydrogenase (LDH) Serum	Assess hepatic, cardiac, renal, muscular or RBC status	Adult: 100–205 mU/ml	

(Continued)

LABORATORY TESTS (cont.)

Test	Purpose	Normal Values	Nursing Actions
Isoenzyme:	Primary source:	% of total:	
LDH 1	heart	24–34%	
LDH 2	heart, erythrocytes	35–45%	
LDH 3	muscle	15–25%	
LDH 4	liver, some muscle	4–10%	
LDH 5	liver, muscle	1–9%	
Leucine aminopeptidase (LAP) Serum	Assess liver, biliary tract, pancreas	1–3 μmole/hr/ml	
Urine		2–18 U/24 hr	Collection container must contain preservative
Lipase Serum	Assess pancreas	0–190 U	Freeze specimen if not done immediately.
Manganese Serum	Assess toxicity	0.4–0.85 mg/ml	
Magnesium (Mg^{++}) Serum	Assess renal, pancreatic, hepatic, thyroid status, Addison's disease	Adult: 1.3–2.5 mEq/L Child: 1.4–1.9 mEq/L Newborn: 1.5–2.3 mEq/L	Alcohol and antacids containing Mg are prohibited for 3 days prior to test
24-hr urine		6.0–8.5 mEq/L	
Parathyroid hormone (PTH) Serum	Assess parathyroid, calcium metabolism	20–70 μL eq/ml	Clients are NPO past midnight prior to test; Specimen is drawn in early AM
Phosphorous (inorganic phosphate, PO_4) Serum	Determine level	Adult: 2.5–4.5 mg/100 ml Child: 3.5–5.8 mg/100 ml	
Porphyrins and porphobilinogens Urine	Assess liver, lead poisoning	50–300 mg/24 hr <2mg/24 hr	Collection container must contain preservative

Test	Purpose	Normal Values	Nursing Actions
Pregnanetriol Urine	Assess adrenal cortex	4mg/24 hr	
Prolactin Serum	Assess pituitary function	Female: 0–23 ng/ml Male: 0–20 ng/ml	Clients are NPO past midnight prior to test; Specimen is drawn in early AM
Protein total Serum	Assess hepatic function, protein altered diseases and dehydration	6–8.1 g/100 ml	
Albumin–globulin ratio (A/G Ratio)		1.5:1 to 2.5:1	
Protein electro-phoresis		Albumin: 3.5–5 g/100 ml Globulin: 2.3–3.5 g/100 ml Alpha 1: 0.1–0.4 g/100 ml Alpha 2: 0.4–1.0 g/100 ml Beta: 0.5–1.1 g/100 ml Gamma: 0.6–1.7 g/100 ml	
Radioactive triolen uptake (I-131 Triolen absorption test)	Assess absorption of bowel and pancreas		
Serum		8–12 % in 4 hr	Client takes I-131-labeled Triolein po; blood samples are drawn at 4, 5, and 6-hr intervals;

(Continued)

LABORATORY TESTS (cont.)

Test	Purpose	Normal Values	Nursing Actions
I-131 Triolen absorbtion test (*cont.*)			
Feces		<2% in 48 hr	Stool is collected for 24 hr; Must be done before any barium testing
Serum glutamicoxaloacetic transaminase (SGOT)	Assess status of many organs, i.e., liver, heart	10–55 nU/ml	
Serum glutamicpyruvic transaminase (SGPT)	Assess status of many organs, especially liver	4–28 mU/ml	
Transferrin Serum	Assess transport of iron	200 mg/100 ml	
Thyroid function Serum	Assess status of thyroid and thyroid disease		
Triiodothyronine (T3 by RIA)		80–205 ng/100 ml	
Free triiodothyronine (FT3)		250–390 pg/100 ml	
Thyroxine (T4)		Adults: 5.0–12.0 μg/100 ml Neonates: 1–5 days: >4.9 μg/100 ml 6–8 days: >4 μg/100 ml 9–11 days: >3.5 μg/100 ml 12–120 days: >3 μg/100 ml	
Free thyroxine (FT4)		1–2.3 ng/100 ml	
Thryoglobulin (Tg)		<50 ng/ml	

Test	Purpose	Normal Values	Nursing Actions
Thyroid function (cont.)			
Thyroxine-binding globulin (TBG)		12–28 μg/ml	
Protein-bound iodine (PBI, butanol-extractable iodine, BEI)		PBI: 4.0–8.0 mg/100 ml BEI: 3.5–6.5 mg/100 ml	Must be done before other tests using iodine media
Thyroid stimulating hormone (TSH)		Adults: 1.9–5.4 μIU/ml Neonates: <25 μIU/ml by 3rd day of life	
Neonatal thyroptropin stimulating hormone		by 3rd day: <25 mIU/ml	
Tubular reabsorption phosphate (TPR) Serum and 24-hr urine	Assess hyperparathyroidism	>78%, assuming balanced dietary intake of Calcium	Client is NPO overnight prior to sample being drawn
Urobilinogen Urine	Assess GI malfunction	Up to 1 mg in a 2–4-hr specimen	Collection container is kept on ice

Please note, these values are guidelines. Check with the laboratory performing the procedure for absolute values.

DRUG LEVELS

Drug	Effective Concentrations
Cimetidine	0.7–3.9 μg/ml
Metronidazole	3–6 μg/ml
Rantidine	100 μg/ml
Tolbutamide	80–240 μg/ml

Please note, these values are guidelines. Check with the laboratory performing the test for absolute values.

GASTRIC ANALYSIS, DIAGNEX BLUE

Gastric analysis is performed to determine the contents of the stomach. A specific consent form may be required.

Nursing Diagnoses for clients undergoing gastric analysis include:

- Alteration in comfort related to procedure
- Anxiety related to procedure
- Knowledge deficit related to diagnostic process

Subjective Data: Client complains of nausea, weight loss, pain, fatigue, or changes in appetite.

Objective Data: Altered physical exam or laboratory findings.

Assessment: Stomach contents are analyzed for acidity, enzymes, cell presence, and response to histamine stimulation. Abnormal results, anacidity or hypersecretion, occur in clients with peptic ulcer, gastritis, pyloric or duodenal obstruction, neoplasms, or pernicious anemia. This procedure uses a nasogastric or salem sump tube to obtain the sample. The Diagnex method, used when only stomach acidity needs to be determined, involves oral ingestion of the dye and a urine specimen collection.

Normal Values:

Fasting residual volume: 20–100 ml
pH: <3.5
Basal acid output (BAO, basal secretion rate): 0–6 mEq/hr
Maximal acid output (MAO, maximal acid output): 10–20 mEq/hr
BAO/MAO ratio: <0.4
Diagnex blue: <6 mg of blue in urine in 2 hours

Nursing Interventions: The procedure is explained to the client. NG tube insertion technique and client participation are discussed. The client is taught to pant if the gag reflex becomes bothersome. The client is prepared to expect a flushed sensation following injection of either Pentagastrin histamine or Histalog betazole hydrochloride. Smoking, which increases gastric motility, is not permitted the day of gastric analysis. Food is withheld for 12 hours and fluid for 8 hours prior to the procedure. If present during this procedure, the nurse provides client reassurance and technical assistance.

Description of the Procedure: This procedure is performed with inpatients and outpatients. The client sits erect while the nasogastric tube is inserted via a nostril and secured with tape. The client reclines and aspiration of the stomach contents takes place. Fifteen to 30 minutes later, stomach contents are aspirated to provide a baseline sample. An IV or IM injection is administered to promote gastric acid secretion. Stomach contents are collected at 15-minute intervals for 2 hours. Blood pressure is monitored frequently to check for hypotension. Other untoward reactions include headache and urticaria. The procedure is completed in approximately 3 hours. The results are available following interpretation.

Evaluating Client Response: The client's gag reflex is assessed. When it is intact, food and medications are then resumed. Client and family support in dealing with the results is provided.

MOTILITY AND CHALLENGE TESTS

- **Motility Tests**
- **Bernstein Test**
- **Glucose Tolerance Test**
- **d-Xylose Absorption–Excretion Test**
- **Pancreatic Secretion Test**
- **Insulin Tolerance Test**
- **Tolbutamide Tolerance Test**
- **Sweat Electrolyte Test**
- **ACTH Stimulation Test**
- **Thyrotropin Releasing Hormone Stimulation Test**

For clients with alterations in nutrition, metabolism, and elimination, diagnostic analysis of digestive and metabolic functions may be needed. Motility studies provide graphic measurement of pressures within the GI tract. Metabolic testing measures breakdown, secretory, or excretory activity. Some procedures require the client to go to the Gastrointestinal (GI) special procedures laboratory, although others can be performed anywhere. A specific consent form may be required for these tests.

Nursing Diagnoses for clients undergoing motility or challenge tests include:

- Alteration in comfort related to procedure
- Anxiety related to procedure
- Knowledge deficit related to diagnostic process

Motility Tests (Esophageal Motility, Anorectal Motility)

Subjective Data: Client complains of dysphagia, heartburn, or regurgitation, constipation or diarrhea.

Objective Data: Abnormal stool analysis and other laboratory values.

Assessment: These tests provide graphic readouts of sphincter pressure. Upper and lower esophageal sphincter pressure is measured and peristalsis quantified; pH can be measured at the same time. Esophageal motility tests are performed on clients who present with complaints regarding swallowing and/or stomach disorders. Anorectal motility studies are performed on clients with unexplained severe constipation or colonic dilation. Pressures within the internal and external anal sphincters are measured.

Nursing Interventions: The procedure is explained to the client. Client cooperation during catheter insertion is explained and encouraged.

Description of the Procedure: This test is performed with inpatients and outpatients. In the GI procedures department, the client undergoing esophageal testing swallows a catheter containing a transducer. The catheter is inserted into the stomach and withdrawn to the level of the sphincters to obtain the manometric pressure readings. An electrode may also be used to measure pH. For anorectal testing, the catheter is inserted via the anus approximately 10 cm into the rectum. The balloon tip is inflated and measurements are made as the catheter is withdrawn. Motility studies take approximately 1 hour to complete. The results are available immediately.

Evaluating Client Response: Client and family support in dealing with the results is provided as needed.

■ Bernstein Test

Subjective Data: Client complains of repeated pain, heartburn, nausea, or vomiting.

Objective Data: A detailed client history and abnormal laboratory values.

Assessment: The Bernstein test is performed to demonstrate the relationship between acid perfusion of the esophageal mucosa and client symptoms, especially pain. A positive result serves as the basis for client treatment.

Nursing Interventions: Client education includes instruction regarding cooperation during tube insertion. The client is told that solutions will be infused via the Levin tube. The specific order and times are not discussed with the client, as test interpretation depends on the client's report of subjective symptoms. Solid foods are not permitted for 3–4 hours prior to this test.

Description of the Procedure: This test is performed with inpatients and outpatients. The client may go to a GI procedures department. The client sits in a chair and a Levin tube is passed via the nares into the stomach. All tubing is draped behind the client so that infusions are changed without client knowledge. Gastric contents are aspirated and the catheter tip is withdrawn to a point 30–35 cm from the nostrils. A control solution of 0.9% NaCl is administered at 120 drops/min for 15 minutes. Subsequently, 0.1% HCl is infused at the same rate for 30 minutes. If the client does not report any pain, the test is considered negative. If the client does report symptoms, the HCl is stopped and 0.9% NaCl administered until all the pain subsides. To be certain that pain is caused by acid perfusion, 0.1% HCl is then readministered. The test is completed and the Levin tube is withdrawn. The client swallows antacid and a glass of milk. The Bernstein test requires approximately $1\frac{1}{2}$ hours to complete. The results are available immediately.

Evaluating Client Response: Following the procedure, the client receives lunch. Further antacid therapy is provided as needed. Client and family support in dealing with the results is provided.

■ Glucose Tolerance Test (GTT, Lactose Tolerance Test, Galactose Tolerance Test, Pentose Tolerance Test)

Subjective Data: Client complains of polyphagia, polydypsia, polyuria, fatigue, abdominal cramping or diarrhea.

Objective Data: Abnormal fasting blood sugar, family history, or multiple yeast infections.

Assessment: A tolerance test is performed to assess the client's ability to metabolize a specific sugar. The results are determined by analyzing venous or capillary whole blood and urine. Glucose tolerance testing is the most frequently performed and is most commonly used to determine if a client has diabetes mellitus. A GTT can also detect adrenal cortical dysfunction, Addison's disease, Simmonds' disease, hyperinsulinism and insulin resistance. Normally, glucose levels peak at 30 minutes after ingestion and approach normal by 2 hours.

Nursing Interventions: Client education includes an explanation of the procedure and preparation for the repeated blood and urine sampling. Some laboratories ask the client to consume a high carbohydrate (150–300 g) diet for 3 days prior to the procedure. All clients are NPO, except for water, past midnight prior to this procedure.

Description of the Procedure: This test is performed with inpatients and outpatients. A venous catheter may be inserted to avoid repeated venipuncture. Capillary whole blood is used in some instances. Baseline blood and urine samples are obtained. The client ingests a test dose of 75 g glucose. It can be given over 3–5 minutes intravenously if needed. Specific dosages for lactose, galactose and pentose tests are available from the laboratory. Blood and urine samples are obtained 30 minutes, 1, and 2 hours after glucose intake. Clients are NPO except for water for the duration of the test. Specimen collection may continue hourly until 5 hours after ingestion. The test is completed after the last blood and urine samples have been obtained. The results are available following interpretation.

Evaluating Client Response: Following the procedure, the client is given lunch. Medication administration is resumed. A positive diagnosis of diabetes mellitus has lifetime implications. Client and family support regarding the results is provided.

■ d-Xylose Absorption–Excretion Test (d-Xylose Tolerance Test)

Subjective Data: Client complains of diarrhea.

Objective Data: Abnormal stool tests and other laboratory values.

Assessment: Xylose, a sugar absorbed solely in the small intestine, does not require pancreatic involvement for digestion. Therefore, impaired absorption and excretion of this sugar indicates the presence of disease in the small intestine. Both blood and urine specimens are collected.

Normal Values:

Urine: >1.2 g in 2 hours
Plasma: 25–40 mg/100 ml in 2 hours

Nursing Interventions: Client education includes an explanation of the procedure. Instructions are provided regarding ingesting the test dose, drinking the required water, and urine collection. Clients are NPO past midnight prior to the procedure.

Description of the Procedure: This test is performed on inpatients and outpatients. Urine collection begins 2 hours before the test dose is administered. The client drinks a test solution containing 5 g to 25 g of d-xylose or a callibrated dose of 10 ml of 5% d-xylose solution per kg of body weight. Plasma levels are drawn 60–120 minutes after ingestion, while urine is collected for an additional 3 hours. No food is allowed during the collection period. The client does drink 3–4 glasses of water during this procedure to maintain urinary output at a minimum of 60 ml/hr. This test requires 5 hours for completion. The results are available following laboratory analysis.

Evaluating Client Response: Following the procedure, the client receives lunch. Medication administration is resumed. Client and family support in dealing with the results is provided.

■ Pancreatic Secretion Test (Secretin Test, Cholecystokinin Test, CCK)

Subjective Data: Client complains of pain, nausea, and vomiting.

Objective Data: Abdominal tenderness, fever, evidence of fluid and electrolyte disturbance, and abnormal laboratory values.

Assessment: This test is used to measure the secretory capacity of the pancreas. Following pancreatic stimulation, duodenal luminal contents are aspirated and analyzed for pancreatic enzyme and secretin. The results indicate the exocrine function of the pancreas. Maximal secretion is normally 2 clinical units of secretin per kilogram body weight and occurs 10–90 minutes after IV injection. Normal bicarbonate concentration is 90 mEq/L.

Nursing Interventions: The procedure is explained to the client and cooperation encouraged. Because this procedure is unpleasant, nursing support of the client is essential. Instructions regarding tube insertion and administration of the test dose are discussed. Clients are NPO past midnight prior to this procedure.

Description of the Procedure: This test is performed with inpatients and outpatients. In the GI procedures department, a mercury-weighted small diameter tube with holes near the tip is passed into the duodenum. Radiographs may be used to determine proper placement. The client either ingests a test meal or receives an IV injection of secretin. Duodenal contents are repeatedly aspirated for up to 2 hours and are kept refrigerated to maintain stability. The tube is then withdrawn and the procedure is complete. A CCK test requires approximately 2 hours for completion. The results are available following laboratory analysis.

Evaluating Client Response: Following the procedure, the client receives lunch. Medication administration is resumed. Client and family support in dealing with the results is provided.

■ Insulin Tolerance Test

Subjective Data: Client complains of anorexia, nausea, abdominal pain, nervousness, headache, or weakness.

Objective Data: Abnormal physical findings including diarrhea, vomiting, weight loss, hyperpigmentation of the skin and mucus membranes, and abnormal data from other laboratory testing.

Assessment: An Insulin Tolerance Test is performed to assess clients with suspected insulin resistance, as in Cushing's syndrome or Acromegaly, Simmonds' disease, Addison's disease, and hyperinsulinism. Normally, glucose levels decrease to 50% of the fasting level by 30 minutes and return to normal in $1\frac{1}{2}$–2 hours.

Nursing Interventions: Client education includes an explanation of the procedure and preparation for repeated blood sampling. The client is asked to consume a high carbohydrate (at least 300 g) diet for 2–3 days prior to the procedure. Clients are NPO past midnight prior to this procedure. Two syringes containing 50 ml 50% Dextrose are kept close in the event a hypoglycemic reaction mandates terminating the test.

Description of the Procedure: This test is performed with inpatients and outpatients. An IV line is inserted to avoid repeated venipuncture. A baseline blood sample is obtained. Regular insulin, 0.1 U/kg of body weight, is then injected intravenously. Blood samples are obtained 20, 30, 45, 60, 90, and 120 minutes following the injection. The results are available following interpretation.

Evaluating Client Response: Following the procedure, the client is given lunch. Medication administration is resumed. The IV line is discontinued unless needed for another reason. Client and family support regarding the results is provided.

■ Tolbutamide Tolerance Test

Subjective Data: Client complains of anorexia, nausea, or fatigue.

Objective Data: Altered physical findings including vomiting, weight loss, altered glucose tests, and other laboratory values.

Assessment: This test is performed to assess clients with suspected islet cell adenomas. Tolbutamide stimulates the production of insulin. Normally, the glucose level is decreased to 50% of the fasting level by 30 minutes and then returns to normal.

Nursing Interventions: Client education includes an explanation of the procedure and preparation for the repeated blood sampling. Clients are NPO past midnight prior to the procedure. Two syringes containing 50 ml 50% Dextrose are kept close by in the event a hypoglycemic reaction mandates terminating the test.

Description of the Procedure: This test is performed on inpatients and outpatients. An IV line or heparin lock is inserted to avoid repeated venipuncture. A baseline venous sample is obtained. Tolbutamide 1.0 g is then injected intravenously over a 2–3 minute period. Blood samples are then obtained 20, 30, 45, 60, 90, and 120 minutes after injection. The results are available following laboratory analysis.

Evaluating Client Response: Following the procedure, the client receives lunch. Medication administration is resumed. Client and family support in dealing with the results is provided.

■ Sweat Electrolyte Test (Iontophoresis Sweat Test)

Subjective Data: Client complains of repeated respiratory infections and diarrhea.

Objective Data: Abnormal physical findings and laboratory values.

Assessment: This test is used to confirm clinical suspicion of cystic fibrosis. It is performed only on children. Sweat chloride >60 mEq/L is diagnostic, whereas 50–60 mEq/L is considered suggestive of cystic fibrosis.

Nursing Interventions: The client is prepared on an age- and developmentally-appropriate level. The families of these children need support in dealing with their child's health, the diagnostic process, and the prognosis. If present during the procedure, the nurse provides encouragement for the child and technical assistance.

Description of the Procedure: This test is performed with inpatients and outpatients. The client's arm is cleaned with water and dried. Two squares of lint soaked in pilocarpine are placed on the flexor surface. A positive electrode is placed on the lint and secured. Two more squares are soaked in magnesium sulphate and placed on the extensor aspect of the same arm. A negative electrode is placed and secured on one of these lints, making certain the two electrodes do not touch. Electrical current is applied and gradually increased. The child may feel some tingling, but it should be mild. After 5 minutes, the current is turned off, electrodes removed, and the forearm cleaned with water and dried. The area where the pilocarpine has been drawn into the skin will appear reddened. Filter paper, held with forceps, is placed on the reddened area and kept in place by strips of polythene and waterproof tape. After 30 minutes, the paper is removed with forceps and sent to the laboratory for analysis. The child's arm is cleaned and dried.

Evaluating Client Response: Postprocedure support for client and family is provided as needed.

■ ACTH Stimulation Test (Cortisol Level, Thorn Test, Dexamethasone Suppression Test, DST)

Subjective Data: Client complains of weakness, fatigue, emotional changes, anorexia, nausea, and vomiting.

Objective Data: Abnormal physical findings including muscle wasting, purple cutaneous striae, ecchymosis, and weight loss.

Assessment: These tests assess adrenal and pituitary gland function by measuring adrenocorticotrophic hormone (ACTH). They are performed on clients with suspected Cushing's syndrome, Addison's disease, adrenal tumor or ACTH-produced tumor elsewhere in the body. A DST is performed to measure increased cortisol activity, whereas an ACTH stimulation test measures decreased cortisol activity.

Normal Values:

Cortisol: 7–9 A.M. = 5–25 μg/100 ml; 4–6 P.M. = 2–13 μg/100 ml
DST: <5μg/100 ml in any sample
ACTH stimulation test: >18 μg/100 ml or 2–3 × baseline value

Nursing Interventions: Nursing actions include client education and preparation regarding these tests. Instructions regarding avoiding undue stress and exercise are provided. The client is told to remain in bed until after the first morning blood specimen has been obtained. NPO status 10–12 hours prior to DST and ACTH stimulation testing is maintained. During these tests, the nurse supports the client by attempting to keep stress levels low. The specimens are placed on ice immediately after drawing to avoid ACTH degradation.

Description of the Procedure: DST and ACTH stimulation tests require overnight hospitalization so the blood sample can be drawn before the client gets out of bed. Cortisol blood levels are drawn by routine venipuncture. The time drawn is included on the requisition. Specific protocols for DST and ACTH tests vary, but general descriptions are as follows. On the previous day, the client undergoing DST receives an IV or IM injection of dexamethasone and is allowed only mild physical activity. The next morning, a blood sample is drawn before the client gets out of bed or eats. The client has a relaxing day and another blood sample is drawn again late in the afternoon. For an ACTH stimulation test, the client is permitted only mild physical activity the day prior. A baseline blood specimen is drawn the morning of the test before the client gets out of bed or eats. The client receives an injection of ACTH either intravenously or intramuscularly. Blood samples are drawn 30 and 60 minutes after injection. These tests involve the client for approximately 24 hours. The results are available following laboratory analysis.

Evaluating Client Response: The venipuncture sites are monitored for bleeding. Client and family support is provided in dealing with the results.

■ Thyrotropin Releasing Hormone Stimulation Test (TRH)

Subjective Data: Client complains of sluggishness, weight gain, sleepiness, and intolerance to cold.

Objective Data: Abnormal physical findings include constipation, menorrhagia, changes in skin and hair, and abnormal results from laboratory tests. Infants may present with persistent physiologic jaundice, hoarse crying, and somnolence.

Assessment: This test is performed to assess the responsiveness of the anterior pituitary gland. It is also used to differentiate between primary, secondary, and tertiary hypothyroidism. Normally, women have higher TSH levels than men and the TSH level increases approximately two times baseline. Maximum response occurs in about 20 minutes.

Nursing Interventions: Client education includes an explanation of the procedure.

Description of the Procedure: The client receives an IV injection of 500 μg of TRH. Blood samples are obtained at intervals of 15–20 minutes for 1–2 hours.

Evaluating Client Response: The client is monitored for inappropriate response to the test dose. Vital signs are monitored and venipuncture sites are checked for bleeding. Client and family support in dealing with the results is provided.

BREATH TESTS

- **Hydrogen Breath Test**
- **Triolein Breath Test**
- **Bile Acid Breath Test**

Breath tests are used to assess gastrointestinal function. GI activity is indirectly monitored by measuring the metabolic breakdown of gases that diffuse across the lumen into the bloodstream and are excreted via the lungs. A specific consent form may be required for these procedures.

Nursing Diagnoses for clients undergoing breath tests include:

- Anxiety related to procedure
- Knowledge deficit related to diagnostic process

Hydrogen Breath Test

Subjective Data: Client complains of pain, nausea, diarrhea, and weight loss.

Objective Data: Abnormal stool analysis and other laboratory values.

Assessment: The hydrogen breath test is a sensitive and highly specific means of testing the intestinal stages of carbohydrate absorption. This test of carbohydrate intolerance is noninvasive and does not use a radioactive isotope. It is, therefore, especially useful in pregnant women and children. When there is maldigestion due to brush border disaccharide deficiency or glucose transport deficit, carbohydrates remain in the intestine and are metabolized by bacteria. The resulting gases, including hydrogen, diffuse readily across the intestine into the bloodstream and are excreted by the lungs. Clients with carbohydrate malabsorption are identified by an increase in hydrogen ion excretion, from the normal of <15 PPM to a diagnostic level of >20 PPM.

Nursing Interventions: The procedure is explained to the client. The noninvasive, nonradioactive nature of this test is emphasized. Instructions concerning exhaling into the collection chamber with lips sealed are provided. Clients are NPO past midnight prior to the exam.

Description of the Procedure: This test is performed with inpatients and outpatients. In the GI procedures department, the client ingests a test solution of carbohydrates. Breath is collected by having the client exhale into a syringe during the late expiratory phase. Measurement takes place 1–3 hours after ingestion. pH is measured. The hydrogen breath test requires approximately 1–3 hours to complete. The results are available following interpretation.

Evaluating Client Response: Following the procedure, food and medications are resumed. Client and family support regarding the results is provided.

■ Triolein Breath Test

Subjective Data: Client complains of pain, nausea, diarrhea, and weight loss.

Objective Data: Abnormal stool analysis and other laboratory values.

Assessment: Triolein breath test, with I-131 labeled triglyceride, had fallen into disuse. Currently, there is interest in performing this test with [C-14]-triolein to identify nonobese clients with maldigestion or malabsorption containing 5 μCi of [C-14]-Triolein, 5 g nonradioactive trioactanoin and dose at their peak collection period.

Nursing Interventions: The procedure is explained to the client. Instructions concerning exhaling with lips sealed into the tube are provided. Clients are NPO past midnight prior to this procedure.

Description of the Procedure: This test is performed with inpatients and outpatients. In the GI procedures department, the client ingests a solution containing 5 μCi of [C-14]-Triolein, 5 g nonradioactive trioactanoin and 30 ml of Lipomul. The client exhales through a tube connected to scintillation fluid that traps the carbon dioxide 3, 4, 5, and 6 hours after ingestion. This fluid is then scanned for radioactivity. The Triolein breath test requires approximately 6 hours to complete. The results are available following interpretation.

Evaluating Client Response: Following the procedure, diet and medications are resumed. Client and family support regarding the results is provided.

■ Bile Acid Breath Test—Biliary Stage

Subjective Data: Client complains of pain, nausea, diarrhea, and weight loss.

Objective Data: Abnormal stool analysis and other laboratory values.

Assessment: The bile acid breath test is a relatively new test for measuring metabolic activity in the intestinal lumen. Normally, ingested conjugated bile acid is absorbed intact in the ileum and recirculated to the liver for excretion. When the client has large quantities of bacteria in the intestine, exposure to these bacteria adversely affects absorption. Using C-14 glycine unconjugated bile acid as a test medium, appreciable amounts of CO_2-14 are released, and diffuse across the gut into the bloodstream. The radioactive CO_2 is then exhaled and can be measured.

Nursing Interventions: The procedure is explained to the client. Instructions concerning exhaling with lips tightly sealed into the tube are provided. Clients are NPO past midnight prior to the exam.

Description of the Procedure: This test is performed with inpatients and outpatients. In the GI procedures department, the client ingests a solution containing C-14-glycine unconjugated bile acids. Following ingestion, the client exhales into a container that traps the carbon dioxide and can be scanned for radioactivity. The bile acid breath test requires 2–4 hours to complete. The results are available following interpretation.

Evaluating Client Response: Following the procedure, diet and medications are resumed. Client and family support regarding the results is provided.

ULTRASONOGRAPHY

Ultrasound is frequently used to examine the biliary tract, liver, and pancreas. Due to the nonechoing quality of air, ultrasound cannot be used for organs that contain air, such as the stomach and intestines. A specific consent form may be required.

Nursing Diagnoses for clients undergoing ultrasound include:

- Alteration in comfort, stomach distension related to procedure
- Anxiety related to procedure
- Knowledge deficit related to diagnostic process

Subjective Data: Client complains of pain, often severe, localized tenderness, rigidity, nausea, fatigue, skin color changes, or increased bleeding.

Objective Data: Abnormal physical findings including ascites or jaundice, vomiting, or altered laboratory values.

Assessment: Ultrasound is the method of choice for visualizing the gall bladder and gallstones and determining if a client will benefit from cholecystectomy. Clients undergoing biliary tract ultrasound either by itself or in conjunction with liver or pancreatic imaging are required to fast overnight to promote gallbladder filling. Biliary ultrasound is performed in the morning to discourage daytime fasting and air swallowing.

Ultrasound of the liver is used to assess clients with suspected focal disease, i.e., cyst, abscess, trauma, or tumor, and suspected diffuse disease, i.e., fatty changes, cirrhosis, acute hepatitis, lymphoma, or leukemia. A comprehensive protocol is required to image all areas of the liver. The dome is especially difficult to visualize due to artifact and transducer angles. Ultrasound is usually performed early in the diagnostic process, since it requires no specific client preparation or x-ray exposure and is highly sensitive and accurate. Ultrasound may also be used as a guide during biopsy.

Ultrasonographic diagnosis in clients with suspected pancreatic disease includes inflammatory disease, neoplasm, pseudocyst formation, or pancreatic phlegma. Concomitant examination is frequently conducted for biliary and pancreatic duct obstruction. To minimize interference from gas within the small bowel, imaging is performed at least 2 hours after the client has eaten or consumed carbonated beverages. To increase the imaging quality of the pancreatic tail, gastric fluid distension may be needed. A fluid intake of as much as 1500 ml may be required. Juices are allowed, but carbonated beverages are prohibited. In addition, imaging may be improved if timed with the respiratory cycle or with different client positions. Ultrasound is also used as a guide when biopsy is performed.

Nursing Interventions: The procedure is explained to the client. Children may require additional assistance during the procedure. Client education includes specific instructions as to fasting and/or fluid intake. Clients are prepared for feeling some pressure during the procedure, changes in position, and cooperating as needed by inhaling or exhaling on request.

Description of the Procedure: Ultrasound is performed with inpatients and outpatients. Privacy is assured. Conductive oil or gel is applied for optimal contact between transducer and skin. The transducer is focused and refocused according to the imaging being performed. The client is asked to inspire deeply and hold his or her breath, and may be asked to do this repeatedly. Ultrasound examinations take approximately 30 minutes to complete. The results are available following interpretation.

Evaluating Client Response: Client and family support regarding the results and potential surgery is provided.

MAGNETIC RESONANCE IMAGING (NUCLEAR MAGNETIC IMAGING, MR, NMR)

MR is a noninvasive method of assessing tissue composition. A specific consent form may be required.

Nursing Diagnoses for clients undergoing MR include:

- Anxiety related to procedure
- Knowledge deficit related to diagnostic process

Subjective Data: Client complains of nausea, anorexia, pain, changes in appetite, or skin changes.

Objective Data: Weight loss or gain, and abnormal physical findings including jaundice or ascites and altered laboratory findings.

Assessment: The use of MR for clients with alterations in nutrition and elimination is increasing as its applications become more clear. MR can examine the temporomandibular joint in clients with facial pain, jaw clicking, locking, or restricted movement. For clients with liver disorders, MR allows the retrohepatic inferior vena cava to be well visualized. Use in clients with pancreatic disease is limited, since it is difficult to visualize the entire pancreas, especially if there is a paucity of retroperitoneal fat. MR is contraindicated in clients with aneurysm clips anywhere in the body or with pacemakers because of the effects of the magnetic field.

Nursing Interventions: Client education includes an explanation of the procedure and the need to remain still during imaging. The ability of the child to cooperate is determined. Sedation and restraints are usually required for infants and young children. Clients are prepared for the imposing size of the MR scanner; the noninvasive nature of the procedure is emphasized. A client health history specific to past insertion of aneurysm clips or pacemaker is obtained. The client changes into a hospital gown and removes all jewelry and prostheses.

Description of the Procedure: This procedure is performed on inpatients and outpatients. The client goes to the MR room. The client is supine within the body scanner during the scanning procedure. Completion time depends upon image quality and may take up to 1 hour. Results are available after interpretation.

Evaluating Client Response: Postprocedure client and family support in dealing with the results is provided as needed.

SCINTIGRAPHY

- Salivary Gland Scan
- Esophageal Scan
- Gastroesophageal Reflux Scan
- Gastric Emptying Scan
- Ectopic Mucosa Scan
- Scintigraphic Gastrointestinal Bleeding Study
- Nonimaging Scintigraphy
- Gall Bladder Scan
- Liver–Spleen Scan
- Pancreas Scan
- Radioactive Iodine Uptake Test
- Thyroid Scan

Many scintigraphic techniques are available to assess pathophysiologic abnormalities of nutrition, metabolism, and elimination. Scintigraphy is used for the many situations in which barium-contrast examinations are contraindicated, nondiagnostic, or normal. Scintigraphy results are quantitative, resulting in accurate evaluation of organ function. A specific consent form may be required for these procedures.

Nursing Diagnoses for clients undergoing scintigraphy include:

- Anxiety related to procedure
- Knowledge deficit related to diagnostic process

Salivary Gland Scan (Parotid Gland Scan)

Subjective Data: Client complains of difficulty swallowing or pain in the neck and/or joints.

Objective Data: Altered physical findings.

Assessment: This scan is performed to determine patency of the salivary and parotid glands. Sjögren's syndrome (in rheumatoid arthritis) can also be assessed. The contrast medium is most commonly IV Tc-99m-sulfur colloid. Scintigraphy is contraindicated during pregnancy and lactation.

Nursing Interventions: The procedure is explained to the client. Potential cross-interference is reduced by allowing 24–48 hours between different nuclear medicine studies. Jewelry, hearing aids, and glasses are removed.

Description of the Procedure: This procedure is performed with inpatients and outpatients. The client is in a sitting position and receives an IV injection of the radioisotope. Scanning begins immediately and continues for 30 minutes. Part way through scanning, the client may be asked to suck on a lemon slice to assess a blocked salivary gland. The entire procedure is completed in less than 30 minutes. The results are available following interpretation.

Evaluating Client Response: Postprocedure support for client and family in dealing with the results is provided.

■ Esophageal Scan

Subjective Data: Client complains of pain or burning.

Objective Data: Altered physical findings.

Assessment: Esophageal scintigraphy is used to quantitate motility abnormalities and gastroesophageal reflux, assess the degree of partial obstruction and determine flow rate. The contrast medium is most commonly oral Tc-99m-sulfur colloid. Scintigraphy is contraindicated during pregnancy and lactation.

Nursing Interventions: The procedure and positioning are explained to the client. Children may need assistance with positioning. Potential cross-interference is reduced by allowing 24–48 hours between different nuclear medicine studies. Retained barium from previous examinations will easily destroy scintigraphic results. Clients are not premedicated with perchlorate. Clients are NPO past midnight prior to this test. Jewelry is removed.

Description of the Procedure: This procedure is performed with inpatients and outpatients. The client assumes a supine position and swallows the Tc-99m-sulfur colloid suspension. Imaging requires 10 minutes for completion. The entire procedure is completed in less than 30 minutes. The esophageal transit time is calculated from the data and is available following interpretation.

Evaluating Client Response: Following the procedure, diet and medications are resumed. Postprocedure support for client and family in dealing with the results is provided.

■ Gastroesophageal Reflux Scan

Subjective Data: Client complains of pain or burning.

Objective Data: Altered physical findings.

Assessment: Suspected gastroesophageal reflux is quantified by means of a radionuclide reflux study. This study is also used to assess client response to therapy. Following ingestion of the contrast medium, water is given to clear the esophagus and to allow motility disturbances to be distinguished from reflux. Binders may be used to apply pressure, and the response measured. The contrast medium is most commonly oral Tc-99m sulfur colloid. Scintigraphy is contraindicated during pregnancy and lactation.

Nursing Interventions: The procedure and positioning are explained to the client. Children may need support as binder pressure is increased and assistance in remaining still during imaging. Potential cross-interference is reduced by allowing 24–48 hours between different nuclear medicine studies. Retained barium from previous examinations will easily destroy scintigraphic results. Clients are not premedicated with perchlorate. The client is NPO past midnight prior to the exam. Jewelry is removed.

Description of the Procedure: This procedure is performed with inpatients and outpatients. First, the client drinks a mixture of orange juice, dilute hydrochloric acid, and Tc-99m-sulfur colloid. The client assumes a supine position and is imaged. The client then drinks water. The binder is applied and esophageal activity is determined at pressures from 0–100 mm Hg in 20-mm Hg increments. The entire procedure is complete in approximately 30 minutes. The results are available following interpretation.

Evaluating Client Response: Following the procedure, diet and medications are resumed. Postprocedure support for client and family in dealing with the results is provided.

■ Gastric Emptying Scan

Subjective Data: Client complains of nausea, fullness, or pain.

Objective Data: Altered physical findings.

Assessment: Gastric emptying scintigraphs involve giving the client a test meal that includes a radionuclide, either Tc-99m or In-111. Test meals vary. Solid meal gastric emptying scintigraphs are more sensitive than liquid meals for detecting abnormalities. More complete assessment of gastric emptying may be acquired by sequential or simultaneous (dual isotope) solid/liquid gastric emptying scintigraphs. The results are expressed either as the percent emptied in 30–60 minutes or as an emptying half-time.

Normal Values: These depend on the type and amount of protein, fat, and carbohydrate in the test meal, since volume and vagal response can alter gastric emptying times. For example, for a solid meal of cooked egg whites, the percent emptied in 60 minutes is 67 + 6%, whereas for a liquid meal of orange juice and normal saline, the percent emptied in 60 minutes is 80 + 10%. Scintigraphy is contraindicated during pregnancy and lactation.

Nursing Interventions: The procedure is explained to the client. Potential cross-interference is reduced by allowing 24–48 hours between different nuclear medicine studies. Retained barium from previous examinations will easily destroy scintigraphic results. Clients are not premedicated with perchlorate. The client is NPO past midnight prior to the exam. Jewelry is removed.

Description of the Procedure: This procedure is performed with inpatients and outpatients. The client ingests the test meal. Imaging is continued until gastric emptying is complete. This procedure is completed in approximately $1\frac{1}{2}$ hours. Results are available following interpretation.

Evaluating Client Response: Following the procedure, diet and medications are resumed. Postprocedure support for client and family in dealing with the results is provided.

■ Ectopic Mucosa Scan (Meckel's Scan)

Subjective Data: Client complains of pain or changes in bowel habits.

Objective Data: Altered physical findings and laboratory tests.

Assessment: Scintigraphy is used to diagnose and/or locate gastric mucosa for clients with suspected Meckel's diverticulum, Barnett's esophagus, or intestinal duplication. Scintigraphy can also distinguish retained antrum from Zollinger–Ellison syndrome. The study is positive for ectopic mucosa if, following IV injection of the radionuclide, a small, "hot" focus appears simultaneously with gastric uptake and bladder activity. Scintigraphy is contraindicated during pregnancy and lactation.

Nursing Interventions: The procedure and its length are explained to the client. Children may need assistance with positioning. Potential cross-interference is reduced by allowing 24–48 hours between nuclear medicine studies. At least 48 hours must elapse between endoscopic or barium examinations and an ectopic mucosa scan. Clients are not premedicated with perchlorate. The client is NPO for 2-8 hours prior to the exam. Jewelry is removed.

Description of the Procedure: This procedure is performed with inpatients and outpatients. The client assumes a supine position and receives an IV injection of the radionuclide. Imaging is performed repeatedly for the first hour. If a suspicious area is noted, imaging is continued over 4 more hours. This procedure takes at least $1\frac{1}{2}$ hours and may take $5\frac{1}{2}$ hours. The results are available following interpretation.

Evaluating Client Response: Following the procedure, diet and medications are resumed. Postprocedure support for client and family in dealing with the results is provided.

■ Scintigraphic Gastrointestinal Bleeding Study

Subjective Data: Client complains of pain or fatigue.

Objective Data: Altered physical findings, including blood in vomitus or stool, and abnormal laboratory data.

Assessment: Scintigraphic gastrointestinal bleeding studies are performed using two different radionuclides and techniques. The resulting scans are examined for unusual "hot" spots. Tc-99m-sulfur colloid studies are considered better for diagnosing active bleeding, whereas studies with Tc-99m-labeled RBC are considered better for diagnosing intermediate bleeding. In the first hour, Tc-99m-labeled RBC studies detect only 15% of abnormalities, but 85% of abnormalities are detected in 24 hours. Scintigraphy is contraindicated during pregnancy and lactation.

Nursing Interventions: The procedure and its length are explained to the client. Children may need assistance in positioning. Since no specific client preparation is required, these studies can be performed on an emergency basis. For nonemergency situations, potential cross-interference is reduced by allowing 24–48 hours between nuclear medicine studies. Retained barium from previous examinations will easily destroy scintigraphic results. Jewelry is removed.

Description of the Procedure: These procedures are performed with inpatients and outpatients. For studies with Tc-99m-sulfur colloid, the client receives the radionuclide by IV injection. Images are obtained every 1–2 minutes for 15 minutes. Additional images are obtained as needed. For Tc-99m-labeled RBC studies, the client is injected intravenously with stannous chloride. After a short interval, a small amount of the client's blood is withdrawn and mixed with Tc-99m-pertechnetate. These cells are reinjected and images obtained every 5 minutes for 30 minutes. Multiple delayed images are obtained for up to 24 hours after the return of the client's labeled RBCs. The initial phase requires approximately 30 minutes to 1 hour, but imaging may be repeated over several hours. The results are available following interpretation.

Evaluating Client Response: Postprocedure support for client and family in dealing with the results is provided as needed.

■ Nonimaging Scintigraphy (In Vivo Scintigraphy)

Subjective Data: Client complains of weakness, fatigue, anorexia, or cramping.

Objective Data: Altered physical findings including changes in stool, and weight loss, and abnormal laboratory data.

Assessment: Nonimaging scintigraphy is used to diagnose and quantitate malabsorption states. Following injection of the radioactive tracer, feces are collected and scanned for that tracer as an indicator of GI tract function. Scintigraphy is contraindicated during pregnancy and lactation.

Nursing Interventions: Client education includes a thorough explanation of the procedure. The importance of including all feces in the collection container is emphasized. Potential cross-interference is reduced by allowing 24–48 hours between nuclear medicine studies. Feces do not require special handling due to the presence of the tracer, but are disposed of in the Nuclear Medicine department.

Description of the Procedure: These procedures are performed with inpatients and outpatients, provided feces can be adequately collected.

GI Blood Loss: Blood is withdrawn from the client, mixed with Cr-51 and injected back into the client. All feces are collected for 3–5 days and then scanned.

Protein Loss: The client receives an IV injection of CrCl-51. This binds to transferrin. Normal feces contain less than 1% CrCl-51 activity in the stool after 4 days.

Steatorrhea: This condition is evaluated by examining the feces following IV injection of C-14-labeled trislein.

Lactose Intolerance: This is determined by examining the feces after the client receives an IV injection of C-14-labeled lactose.

Evaluating Client Response: Postprocedure support for client and family in dealing with the results is provided as needed.

■ Gall Bladder Scan (Tc-99m-Cholescintigraphy, DISIDA Scan)

Subjective Data: Client complains of pain.

Objective Data: Altered physical findings including tenderness to percussion and jaundice.

Assessment: Currently, the use of Technetium Diisopropyl-Iminodiacetic Acid-99m (DISIDA) scintigraphy is so widespread that a procedure with significant false-positive results and a high incidence of contrast reactions, IV cholangiography, has been virtually eliminated. A normal Tc-99m-cholescintigram demonstrates, within 1 hour, rapid biliary excretion with gallbladder filling and duodenal activity. Failure of the gall bladder to visualize within 4 hours is abnormal and suggestive of acute cholecystitis. Fasting prior to the procedure is essential so that the gall bladder does not contract during isotope excretion and thus prevent the tracer from entering the gall bladder. Scintigraphy is contraindicated during pregnancy and lactation.

Nursing Interventions: The procedure is explained to the client. Children may need assistance in remaining still. Potential cross-interference is reduced by allowing 24–48 hours between different nuclear medicine studies. This study must be completed before any barium testing. The client is NPO for at least 4 hours prior to the exam. Jewelry is removed.

Description of the Procedure: This procedure is performed with inpatients and outpatients. The client reclines and receives an IV injection of Tc-99m-DISIDA. Imaging is performed 1 hour after injection. If the gallbladder does not visualize, imaging may be repeated 2–6 hours after injection. The client remains NPO until imaging is completed. This procedure takes 1–6 hours to complete. Repeat images are sometimes obtained 24 hours after injection. The results are available following interpretation.

Evaluating Client Response: Following the procedure, diet and medications are resumed. Postprocedure support for client and family in dealing with the results is provided.

Liver–Spleen Scan (Liver Scan)

Subjective Data: Client complains of malaise, fatigue, and weight loss.

Objective Data: Altered physical findings including jaundice, ascites and skin changes, and abnormal laboratory data.

Assessment: Liver spleen scans are performed using Tc-99m-sulfur colloid. This Tc-99m-labeled iminodiacetic derivative has replaced I-131-Rose Bengal as the radionuclide of choice for liver scintigraphy. Tc-99m-labeled sulfur colloid is picked up by the Kupffer cells for excretion. Imaging detects those areas of the liver devoid of Kupffer cells and examines splenic anatomy. Various pathophysiologic states are determined according to differing patterns of tracer uptake. Heterogeneous uptake occurs in clients with cirrhosis, hepatitis, and diffuse infiltrative processes, both benign and malignant. Solitary lesions visualized include cysts, hematomas, hemangiomas, abscesses, adenomas, and solitary metastasis. Multiple, well-circumscribed lesions are seen in metastases to the liver. Using the gamma camera computer, functional imaging of the liver can determine time activity curves for measurement of blood clearance, maximal hepatic uptake, liver clearance, and liver transit time. Liver–spleen scans are also used to determine the cause of existing jaundice. Scintigraphy is contraindicated during pregnancy and lactation.

Nursing Interventions: The procedure is explained to the client. Potential cross-interference is reduced by allowing 24–48 hours between different nuclear medicine studies. Liver spleen studies are completed before, or at least 24 hours after, any barium procedures. Abdominal x-rays may be obtained to determine client readiness for liver spleen scanning after barium testing. Children are frequently NPO prior to this test and may need assistance with positioning. Jewelry is removed.

Description of the Procedure: This procedure is performed with inpatients and outpatients. The client reclines and receives an IV injection of Tc-99m-sulfur colloid. Imaging is performed and is repeated over approximately 2 hours. The results are available following interpretation.

Evaluating Client Response: Following the procedure, food and medications are resumed. Postprocedure support for client and family in dealing with the results is provided as needed.

Pancreas Scan

Subjective Data: Client complains of pain, anorexia, nausea, and vomiting.

Objective Data: Altered physical findings including jaundice, weight loss, abnormal stools, and altered laboratory data.

Assessment: Pancreas scans reveal the size and position of the pancreas, in addition to demonstrating the presence of malignancy, obstructive jaundice, and pancreatitis. Selenomethionine is the radioisotope currently in use. The pancreas visualizes with relative difficulty due to the larger mass of the adjacent liver. Scintigraphy is contraindicated during pregnancy and lactation.

Nursing Interventions: The procedure is explained to the client and the importance of remaining still is emphasized. Children may require assistance with positioning. Detailed instructions regarding the required dietary intake is provided. Potential cross-interference is reduced by allowing 24–48 hours between different nuclear medicine studies. Jewelry is removed.

Description of the Procedure: Pancreas scans are performed with inpatients and outpatients. The client eats a low-fat supper the prior evening and a normal breakfast 30 minutes before the procedure. The client may receive an injection of morphine to constrict the sphincter of Odi, or urecholine to stimulate tracer uptake. The radioisotope is administered intravenously. Imaging begins immediately and continues for up to 1 hour with the client in the same still position. The results are available following interpretation.

Evaluating Client Response: Postprocedure support for client and family in dealing with the results is provided as needed.

■ Radioactive Iodine Uptake Test (RAIU, Radioactive Iodine Thyroid Scan)

Subjective Data: Client complains of malaise, fatigue, and weight loss.

Objective Data: Altered physical findings, including skin, nail and hair changes, and abnormal laboratory data.

Assessment: Radioactive iodine uptake testing is performed to assess functioning and pathology of the thyroid gland. Following oral administration of a test dose of I-131, the uptake percentage is calculated. This procedure is frequently combined with thyroid imaging. Results are significantly affected by the client's intake of iodide or thyroid hormone. Scintigraphy is contraindicated during pregnancy and lactation.

Normal Values:
1%–3% absorbed after 2 hours
2%–25% absorbed after 6 hours
15%–45% absorbed after 24 hours

Nursing Interventions: The procedure is explained to the client and the importance of remaining still is emphasized. Children may require assistance with positioning. A detailed client history regarding iodine and thyroid hormone intake (using both generic and trade names) is obtained. Clients are asked specific questions about intake of Lugol's solution, potassium iodide or other inorganic iodides, and intake of seafood within the previous 2 weeks. Clients are also questioned about any contrast studies they may ever have undergone. Estrogen therapy is questioned, as estrogen may cause false high readings. Jewelry is removed.

Description of the Procedure: These procedures are performed with inpatients and outpatients. On day 1, the client ingests the radioactive tracer in pill form. Imaging is performed 24 hours later with the client in a supine position holding the neck still. Repeat uptakes may be obtained during the next 24 hours. This procedure takes approximately 15 minutes for imaging each time. The results are available following interpretation.

Evaluating Client Response: Postprocedure support for client and family in dealing with the results is provided as needed.

■ Thyroid Scan

Subjective Data: Client complains of malaise, fatigue, and weight changes.

Objective Data: Altered physical findings including skin, nail and hair changes, and abnormal laboratory data.

Assessment: Thyroid scans are performed to assess location, size, shape, and anatomical function for clients with clinical evidence of substernal or enlarged thyroid glands. Clients present with symptoms associated with hyperthyroidism, hypothyroidism, or Graves disease. An area of thyroid nonfunction may lead to further investigation for the presence of malignancy. I-131 has been the most commonly used radioisotope; however, I-125 and sodium pertechnetate-99m are also used. Scintigraphy is contraindicated during pregnancy and lactation.

Nursing Interventions: The procedure is explained to the client and the need to remain still without coughing or swallowing is emphasized. Children may require assistance to remain still. Using both generic and trade names, a detailed client history regarding iodine and thyroid hormone intake is obtained. Clients are asked specific questions about intake of Lugol's solution, potassium iodide, or other inorganic iodides, and intake of seafood within the previous 2 weeks. Clients are also questioned about any contrast studies they may ever have undergone. Estrogen therapy is questioned, as estrogen may cause false-high readings. Thyroid medications, oral contraceptives, and vitamins may be withheld for several days prior to this procedure. Jewelry is removed.

Description of the Procedure: This procedure is performed with inpatients and outpatients. The client goes to the Nuclear Medicine Department and receives an IV injection of radioisotope. Imaging is performed with the client in a supine position, with the neck stabilized. This procedure takes approximately 1 hour to complete. Imaging may be repeated in 3–6 hours and again in 24 hours. The results are available following interpretation.

Evaluating Client Response: Postprocedure support for client and family in dealing with the results is provided as needed.

RADIOLOGY

- **Dental x-rays**
- **Abdominal x-rays**

Radiographs are a cornerstone of diagnosis for oral health and a baseline for assessing the abdomen. A specific consent form may be required for these procedures.

Nursing Diagnoses for clients undergoing x-rays include:

- Anxiety related to procedure
- Knowledge deficit related to diagnostic process

Dental X-Rays (Temperomandibular Joint (TMJ) Arthrotomograms)

Subjective Data: Client complains of pain.

Objective Data: May be negative or include altered physical findings of swelling, erythema or clicks.

Assessment: X-rays are used to assess bone and tooth structure and the presence of dental caries, cysts, abcesses or neoplasms within the mouth. In children and adolescents, unerupted permanent teeth are visualized. Cephalometric x-rays are taken to determine tooth formation and jaw structure. X-rays are also used to determine the extent of facial trauma and the need for surgical correction. TMJ tomograms focus on one plane of the joint while blurring others. Arthrotomograms allow for analysis of bone structure and demonstrate the relationship of bone to soft tissues such as vascular and connective tissue.

Nursing Interventions: Client education includes an explanation of the procedure with emphasis on remaining still.

Description of the Procedure: This procedure is performed with inpatients and outpatients. Clients are positioned in the dental chair and draped with a lead apron and/or thyroid collar to prevent exposure to scatter radiation. For some dental x-rays the film is placed in the client's mouth and the client is instructed to bite gently and remain still. The camera is positioned relative to the client. Panoramic x-rays are obtained by a camera that circles the client's head. For tomograms the client may be asked to keep the mouth partially opened. Dental x-rays are complete in less than 5 minutes. The results are available following interpretation.

Evaluating Client Response: Postprocedure client and family support is provided.

■ Abdominal X-Rays (Flat Plate)

Subjective Data: Client complains of pain, nausea, fullness or diarrhea.

Objective Data: Findings include altered physical exam or laboratory data.

Assessment: Abdominal x-rays are used to assess the size, shape and position of abdominal organs and to determine the presence of gas, ascites or obstruction. Abdominal x-rays do not require contrast medium and are frequently the first radiologic procedure performed in the diagnostic process. Abdominal x-rays are contraindicated during pregnancy.

Nursing Interventions: The procedure is explained to the client. Scheduling takes into account that abdominal x-rays may be ineffective if they follow barium or other ingested or rectally inserted contrast medium procedures. All jewelry is removed and the client wears a hospital gown.

Description of the Procedure: This procedure is performed with inpatients and outpatients. The client stands and is positioned relative to the camera. The client may be asked to inspire and hold a deep breath. This test takes less than 5 minutes. The results are available following interpretation.

Evaluating Client Response: Postprocedure support for client and family is provided as they deal with the need for further diagnostic testing.

COMPUTED TOMOGRAPHY (COMPUTERIZED AXIAL TOMOGRAPHY, CT, CAT SCAN, EMI)

Computed tomography is used to examine clients with alterations in nutrition, metabolism, and elimination. CT is as effective as sonography for hepatic or biliary disease, but is used less frequently, since it exposes the client to ionizing radiation and is more expensive. A specific consent form is required.

Nursing Diagnoses for clients undergoing CT include:

- Anxiety related to procedure
- Knowledge deficit related to diagnostic process
- Potential for injury: allergic reaction related to procedure

Subjective Data: Client complains of pain, localized tenderness, rigidity, nausea, fatigue, weakness, skin color changes, or increased bleeding.

Objective Data: Altered physical findings including ascites or jaundice, vomiting, or abnormal laboratory data.

Assessment: CT is used for clients with many different suspected pathophysiologies. For clients with suspected temporomandibular joint (TMJ) dysfunction, CT can identify trauma, tumor, and derangements of the joint. The gastrointestinal tract can be examined for masses, polyps, etc. For clients with biliary disease, CT may be used to identify biliary obstruction and the level at which it occurs. CT can be used to differentiate normal and abnormal adrenal glands.

Liver CT scans require a comprehensive protocol, as visualization of the dome of the liver is affected by the variable depths of inspiration. CT is effective in identifying the distribution of lesions, the extent of primary tumor, and the presence of diffuse fatty infiltration or hemochromatosis. CT is used to assess the potential for surgical segmental resection in clients with hepatoma.

Clients with acute pancreatitis may undergo contrast-enhanced CT scans to determine potential complications, especially pseudocyst formation and development of pancreatic phlegma. This scan requires the administration of contrast medium. CT may also be used as a guide during percutaneous aspiration. CT is preferred in the diagnosis of suspected neoplasm because it permits visualization of the entire gland, including the pancreatic tail.

Nursing Interventions: Client education includes an explanation of the procedure and the need to remain completely still during imaging. The ability of the child to lie still and/or the need for sedation or restraint of the very young child is determined. Clients are prepared for the imposing size of the CT scanner and the noninvasive nature of the procedure is emphasized. If the client is undergoing a contrast-enhanced scan, a history specific for pregnancy, allergy to iodine, or previous reaction to contrast medium is elicited. Scheduling considerations for clients undergoing multiple diagnostic studies are essential. The barium or iodine oral-contrast preparations used for CT scanning are intentionally less dense than those used in other radiologic examinations. Residual barium from other examinations will destroy the CT image, but residual barium from CT scanning will not impair others. Clients are frequently NPO 2–4 hours prior to CT, especially for contrast-enhanced scans. Clear liquids are sometimes permitted. The client changes into a hospital gown, removes all jewelry and prostheses, voids, and goes to the CT room.

Description of the Procedure: CT scanning is performed with inpatients and outpatients. For TMJ imaging, the client's mouth may be packed with gauze or a bite splint to eliminate movement during scanning. Virtually all abdominal CT scanning is contrast enhanced in order to distinguish unopacified fluid-filled bowel loops from abdominal masses. Flavored, low-density barium preparations have been developed for CT use. For abdominal CT scans, the client drinks the contrast medium, whereas the contrast medium is injected intravenously for hepatic or biliary scanning. Administration of contrast medium may precede scanning by up to 1 hour. The client is supine within the body scanner during the scanning procedure. The client is told to lie still and may be asked to inspire and hold a deep breath. This procedure is completed in less than 30 minutes. Results are available after interpretation.

Evaluating Client Response: Diet and medications are resumed. Fluid intake is encouraged to assist in eliminating the oral contrast medium. Postprocedure client and family support in dealing with the results is provided.

CONTRAST STUDIES

- **Temporomandibular Joint Arthrography**
- **Upper Gastrointestinal Study**
- **Lower GI Series**
- **Percutaneous Transhepatic Cholangiography**
- **Angiography**

Using various contrast media and insertion techniques, many different contrast studies are performed with clients who are experiencing alterations in nutrition or elimination. A specific consent form is required for these procedures.

Nursing Diagnoses for clients undergoing contrast studies include:

- Alteration in comfort related to procedure
- Alteration in elimination related to procedure
- Anxiety related to diagnostic process
- Knowledge deficit related to procedure
- Potential for injury: allergic reaction related to procedure

■ Temporomandibular Joint Arthrography (TMJ Arthrogram)

Subjective Data: Client complains of pain.

Objective Data: Clicking or locking of the TMJ.

Assessment: TMJ arthrograms are indicated for clients with clinical evidence of internal derangement of the soft tissues of this joint. The relationship between hard tissue, i.e., bone, and soft tissue—disc, vascular, and connective tissue—is examined. The position, dynamics, and integrity of the meniscus are assessed. Extreme caution is used in clients with prior allergic reaction to contrast medium. Caution is also required for clients with acute infection of the articular area or other regional infections including otitis media and parotid gland infection.

Nursing Interventions: The procedure is explained to the client. Children may require assistance to remain still. The client is prepared to expect some postprocedure discomfort. Clients are NPO 2–4 hours prior to the procedure. Instructions are provided regarding postprocedure analgesics and diet. A client history specific for prior reaction to contrast medium or allergy to iodine is obtained. The client removes all prostheses and jewelry.

Description of the Procedure: This procedure is performed in a radiology area with inpatients and outpatients. The client reclines with the head firmly supported by the radiology table and with the affected side up. The preauricular area is located and prepared. Local anesthesia is injected into the soft tissues and then deeper into the joint space. The client is asked to open and close the mouth while fluoroscopy is used to locate the desired entry area into the joint space. The eyeblink reflex is assessed frequently. If this reflex is sluggish from the local anesthetic, the eyelid is taped closed to prevent corneal damage. Under fluoroscopic guidance, a catheter is inserted into the joint space. The water-soluble contrast medium is inserted and the angiocath withdrawn. Radiographs and/or tomograms are obtained quickly, since the contrast medium starts to disperse 10–15 minutes after injection. After the radiographic portion is complete, pressure is applied to the joint space with sterile gauze and an icepack. This procedure is completed in 1 hour. The results are available following interpretation.

Evaluating Client Response: The entry site is assessed for bleeding or excessive swelling. Some swelling and moderate discomfort, especially upon opening, are expected. Analgesics are administered as needed. The client resumes eating with a full liquid or dental soft diet and increases to a regular diet as tolerated.

■ Upper Gastrointestinal Study (Upper GI, Barium Swallow, Small Bowel Series, Double Contrast, Enteroclysis)

Subjective Data: Client complains of pain, cramping, dysphagia, dyspepsia, anorexia, "gas," or fatigue.

Objective Data: The presence of abnormal stools, weight loss, and abnormal findings on physical and laboratory testing.

Assessment: An upper GI series is used to assess a client with evidence of esophageal varices, gastric spasm, ulcerations, malignant infiltrate, or other anatomic abnormalities. The presence of celiac disease, regional enteritis, or malabsorption syndrome can also be assessed. Following oral ingestion of insoluble radiopaque contrast medium, serial fluoroscopy and exposed radiographs are used to examine the esophagus, stomach, pyloric valve, and duodenum. Single contrast studies are preferred for evaluation of peristalsis and wall motion, although double contrast studies (air inserted for further contrast) are preferred for visualization of mucosal detail and evaluation of distensibility. Upper GI studies may also be performed with small bowel follow-through and may include biopsy. Enteroclysis allows the radiologist greater control of the contrast medium. For this procedure, a tube is passed via the nose or mouth and advanced to the jejunum. The contrast medium is then inserted at varying rates via the tube. Enteroclysis can be performed as either a single contrast or double contrast study. An upper GI series is contraindicated for clients with suspected colonic obstruction, due to the potential for barium impaction.

Nursing Interventions: The procedure, preparation, and follow-up care are explained to the client. Children may need special encouragement to swallow the contrast medium and to remain still during the procedure. Bowel preparation prior to an upper GI series varies with the institution. Some clients may be placed on low-residue and/or clear-liquid diets prior to the procedure. To promote GI emptying, clients receive laxatives, cathartics and/or enemas the night before and/or the morning of the test. Children receive age-appropriate bowel preparation. Clients are NPO for 12 hours prior to an upper GI. Smoking, which stimulates gastric motility, is discouraged. Alcohol is not permitted for 24 hours prior to the procedure. The client is prepared for swallowing the contrast medium and for position changes during the procedure. If performed on an outpatient basis, the client must be willing and able to comply with the preprocedure protocol. Scheduling takes into account that CT, ultrasonography, and scintigraphy studies are easily destroyed by retained barium. For female clients, the possibility of pregnancy must be excluded. The client wears a hospital gown, removes all jewelry, and voids prior to the procedure.

Description of the Procedure: This procedure is performed with inpatients and outpatients. In the radiology department, the client swallows approximately 300–600 cc of contrast medium. Its progress through the GI tract is followed by means of fluoroscopy and serial, timed radiographs. Initially, the client stands, but changes position for follow-up imaging. If gastric emptying and small bowel motility need to be assessed, follow-up radiographs may be obtained over 24 hours. When double contrast studies are obtained, the client first ingests the thick barium sulfate solution and then swallows tablets that release carbon dioxide in the GI tract. The initial phase of an upper GI series takes 2–6 hours, depending on individual client need. Preliminary results may be available immediately, but definitive diagnosis follows interpretation.

Evaluating Client Response: Following the procedure, diet and medications are resumed. The client is encouraged to drink large amounts of fluid to promote barium excretion and prevent impaction. Passage of barium in the stool is recorded. Client and family support in dealing with the results is provided.

■ Lower GI Series (Barium Enema, BE, Double Contrast)

Subjective Data: Client complains of pain, cramping, or constipation.

Objective Data: The presence of abnormal stools and abnormal findings on physical and laboratory testing.

Assessment: During a lower GI, radiopaque contrast medium is inserted rectally, or via a stoma if present, into the client and followed by fluoroscopy and serial timed radiographs. The contour of the entire colon including cecum and appendix is examined. Single contrast studies are used to evaluate obstruction, diverticuli and ischemia. Double contrast studies, which use more radiation, require denser barium and greater client cooperation, demonstrate the mucosa in detail. Double contrast studies are preferred for examining polyps, small nonobstructing carcinomas, or inflammatory bowel disease. This procedure is contraindicated for clients with toxic megacolon. Extreme caution is necessary if this procedure is required for clients with severe inflammatory bowel disease. In addition, caution is required when performing this procedure on clients with a known history of cardiac dysrhythmia.

Nursing Interventions: The procedure, preparation, and postprocedure care are explained. Children may require assistance with positioning during the procedure. The client is prepared for rectal insertion of the contrast medium and for position changes during the procedure. Adequate bowel preparation is essential. Repeat testing increases cost, time, client participation, and radiation exposure. Fecal bulk is reduced by placing the client on a low-residue or clear-liquid diet for 2–3 days prior to a lower GI. Fluid intake should, however, be increased. Laxatives and/or suppositories are administered. The client receives enemas until clear prior to the test. Enema technique is important. Numerous small enemas cleanse the rectosigmoid but leave the right colon unprepared. A 2-liter enema is needed to cleanse this area. Children receive age-appropriate bowel preparation. Clients are NPO for 8–12 hours prior to this test. If performed on an outpatient basis, the client must be willing and able to comply with the preprocedure protocol. Scheduling takes into account that upper GI, CT, sonography, scintigraphy and excretory urography studies are easily destroyed by retained barium and should be completed before BE. For female clients, the possibility of pregnancy must be excluded. The client wears a hospital gown, removes all jewelry and prostheses, and voids prior to the procedure.

Description of the Procedure: This procedure is performed with inpatients and outpatients. In the radiology department, the client is positioned on the left side and a rectal tube is inserted. For some clients, a

French catheter with balloon is used to prevent barium excretion before the test is completed. The contrast medium is inserted. Client position may then change depending on the areas to be examined. Fluoroscopy and serial timed radiographs are obtained. Follow-up radiographs may be obtained following evacuation of the contrast medium or 24 hours later. Air contrast studies, with air inserted through the rectal tube are sometimes used to detect finer details. Glucagon may be administered to promote colonic relaxation and to allow adequate distension of the bowel without spasms. Lower GI series are complete in 1–2 hours. Preliminary results may be available immediately, but definitive diagnosis follows interpretation.

Evaluating Client Response: Following this procedure, the client receives evacuating enemas and/or laxatives. Food and medications are resumed. The client is encouraged to drink large amounts of fluid to promote barium excretion and prevent impaction. The passage of barium in the stool is noted. This procedure can produce significant fatigue. A postprocedure rest period is provided. Client and family support in dealing with the results is provided.

■ Percutaneous Transhepatic Cholangiography (PTC)

Subjective Data: Client complains of pain or itching.

Objective Data: The presence of jaundice and other abnormal findings on physical exam and laboratory testing.

Assessment: PTC is used to locate the site of obstruction in jaundiced clients. This procedure is the result of development of the Chiba needle, a "skinny" needle that allows penetration of the intrahepatic bile ducts. The needle is inserted into the liver and very slowly withdrawn until radiopaque contrast medium can be seen filling the dilated biliary system above the level of obstruction. Clients undergoing this procedure often also undergo endoscopic retrograde cholangiopancreaticography.

Nursing Interventions: The procedure and the importance of remaining still are explained to the client. Children may need assistance in positioning during the procedure. A client history specific for previous reaction to contrast medium or allergy to iodine is obtained. Laboratory testing to determine clotting status is performed. For female clients, the possibility of pregnancy must be excluded. The client is NPO past midnight prior to the procedure. Scheduling takes into account that previous barium studies may impair visualization. The client wears a hospital gown, removes all jewelry and prostheses, and voids prior to the procedure.

Description of the Procedure: This procedure is performed with inpatients and outpatients. The adequacy of the client's clotting status is determined. In the radiology department, the client is positioned for percutaneous injection into the liver. The entry site is determined and prepared. The needle is inserted and, via fluoroscopy, the position of the needle in the liver is determined. The needle is withdrawn very slowly as the contrast medium is inserted. When filling of the biliary tree occurs, serial radiographs are obtained. The needle is withdrawn and the entry site checked for signs of bleeding. PTC may be completed in 1–2 hours. Preliminary results may be available immediately, but definitive diagnosis follows interpretation.

Evaluating Client Response: Vital signs are monitored and the entry site is checked for bleeding. Food and medications are resumed. Fluid intake is encouraged to promote excretion of the contrast medium. If an obstruction is visualized, surgery may be performed soon after completion of PTC. The client and family are prepared for this possibility.

■ Angiography

Subjective Data: Client complains of nausea, anorexia, pain, or change in bowel habits.

Objective Data: The presence of abnormal findings on physical exam and other diagnostic testing.

Assessment: Clients with alterations in nutrition or elimination may undergo angiography of the mesentery, pancreas, liver, or spleen. Angiography is performed to assess circulation and the presence and nature of masses. Contrast medium is inserted into the desired area and serial radiographs obtained. Due to the risk inherent in entering a blood vessel, especially an artery, other procedures precede angiography in the diagnostic process.

Nursing Interventions: The procedure, the need to remain still, and post-procedure monitoring are explained to the client. The ability of the child to cooperate and the need for sedation or restraints is determined. The client is told that injection of the contrast medium may provoke an unpleasant feeling. A client history specific for pregnancy and for prior allergic response to contrast medium is obtained. Adequacy of clotting status is determined. Anticoagulant therapy may be temporarily interrupted. The client is NPO past midnight prior to the procedure. The client wears a hospital gown and removes all jewelry and prostheses, and voids prior to the procedure.

Description of the Procedure: This procedure is performed with inpatients and outpatients when sufficient postprocedure monitoring is available. In the x-ray room, the entry site is prepared. Local anesthesia is administered and the entry site draped. The client is instructed not to move until the test is complete. A catheter is inserted and threaded via fluoroscopy to the desired site. Contrast medium is inserted through the catheter and serial timed radiographs obtained. Many clients report discomfort associated with catheter manipulation or contrast insertion during this procedure. The catheter is withdrawn. Sutures or dressings may be applied to the entry site. This procedure takes approximately 1–2 hours. Preliminary results may be available immediately, but final interpretation follows detailed viewing of the films.

Evaluating Client Response: Following the procedure, the client is kept supine with the entry site immobilized. Pressure, by sandbag or dressing, may be applied. The insertion site is checked for signs of bleeding. Arterial pulses, skin color, and temperature distal to the insertion site are closely monitored. Vital signs are taken every 15 minutes the first hour, every 30 minutes for the next 2 hours, and every 4 hours prn. Food and medications are resumed. Fluid intake is encouraged to promote excretion of the contrast medium. Pain medication may be offered. Client and family support in dealing with the results is provided.

DIRECT VISUALIZATION

- **Upper Gastrointestinal Fiberoscopy**
- **Colonoscopy**
- **Anoscopy**
- **Endoscopic Retrograde Cholangiopancreaticography**

Direct visualization of the gastrointestinal tract can be achieved via the mouth, anus, or stoma, if present. In addition, fiberoptic scopes also permit photography, tissue biopsy, and minor surgical repair. Due to the invasive nature of these procedures, they may follow other preliminary tests. Direct visualization does, however, precede barium studies. A specific consent form is required for these procedures.

Nursing Diagnoses for clients undergoing direct visualization include:

- Alteration in comfort related to procedure
- Anxiety related to procedure
- Knowledge deficit related to diagnostic process
- Potential difficulty in swallowing related to procedure

Upper Gastrointestinal Fiberoscopy (Endoscopy, Esophagoscopy, Gastroscopy)

Subjective Data: Client complains of dysphagia, anorexia, fatigue, change in bowel habits, or pain.

Objective Data: Weight loss, vomiting, altered physical findings, and abnormal blood or stool analyses.

Assessment: Esophagoscopy and gastroscopy provide direct visualization of the upper gastrointestinal tract through a flexible fiberoptic endoscope. They are performed to assess clients with suspected gastritis, gastric ulcer, esophageal or gastric mass, hemorrhage or obstruction. Due to scope size limitations, this procedure is performed less frequently with children than with adults.

Nursing Interventions: The procedure is explained and the client is prepared for swallowing the endoscope and its movement during the procedure. Postprocedure monitoring is also explained. This procedure must be performed prior to any barium studies. If biopsy is performed during endoscopy, follow-up barium studies are delayed for 3 days. When performed on a scheduled basis, clients are NPO past midnight prior to endoscopy. An IV line may be established for medication administration prior to and during the procedure. A sedative and/or narcotic are administered prior to the procedure. To dry secretions, atropine may also be given. Appropriate precautions, such as raising side rails after giving sedatives or narcotics, are observed. All client prostheses are removed. If present during the procedure, the nurse provides client reassurance and technical assistance.

Description of the Procedure: These procedures are performed with inpatients and outpatients and may be performed bedside. To achieve local anesthesia of the pharynx, either the client gargles with lidocaine or the lidocaine is sprayed on the pharynx. The fiberoptic endoscope is inserted through the mouth. A mouth guard may be used to protect the client, endoscope, and endoscopist from injury due to biting. Position of the endoscope may be changed frequently during the procedure by maneuvers such as rotation, pulling back, or further insertion. When the procedure is complete, the endoscope and mouth guard are withdrawn. Length of time for the procedure depends on what is specifically involved and ranges from 10 minutes to about 1 hour. The results of visualization are available immediately; results of biopsies or other tests requiring laboratory analysis take longer to obtain.

Evaluating Client Response: Following the procedure, vital signs are monitored and the client closely observed for dyspnea. If any excision was performed, some blood may be expected in emesis or stool. Otherwise, bleeding is considered an adverse reaction and the physician is notified. The client is NPO until return of the gag reflex, which is determined by a light touch of a tongue blade to the uvula. This may take several hours, depending on the sedation and anesthesia used. Oral intake then begins with sips of water or ice chips. Close monitoring is maintained to be certain the client swallows with no difficulty. Food and medications are then resumed. Since cramping of the gastrointestinal musculature frequently occurs, clients often complain of discomfort. Analgesia is administered as needed. Postprocedure client and family support in dealing with the results is provided.

■ Colonoscopy (Flexible Sigmoidoscopy, Rectosigmoidoscopy)

Subjective Data: Client complains of change in bowel habits, pain, or fatigue.

Objective Data: Altered physical findings and abnormal laboratory blood or stool analyses.

Assessment: Examination of the left, transverse, and right colon, as well as the sigmoid is performed with a flexible fiberoptic endoscope inserted via the anus. Colonoscopy is used to assess clients with melena, persistent diarrhea, suspected mucosal inflammation or ulceration, hemorrhage, or carcinoma. Polyps located during endoscopic exam can be removed at that time.

Nursing Interventions: The procedure and preparation are explained. The ability of the child to cooperate and the need for additional sedation or restraint is determined. Instructions include bowel preparation, enema technique, and medications and their side effects. The client is prepared for insertion of the scope, its movement, and insertion of air. Scheduling takes into account that this procedure must be performed prior to any barium studies. If biopsy is to be performed during colonoscopy, follow-up barium studies should be delayed for 3 days. Better visualization is achieved when the bowel is empty. Bowel preparation varies with the institution. A clear-liquid diet may be ordered for 1–3 days prior to the exam. Clients are NPO overnight in advance of this procedure. Cathartics may be administered 24–48 hours before the exam and suppositories or enemas administered the night before and 1–2 hours prior to the exam. Sedatives and/or narcotics are administered orally or intramuscularly prior to and intravenously during the procedure to promote client relaxation and reduce muscle spasm. Appropriate precautions, such as raising side rails after giving sedatives or narcotics, are observed. All prostheses are removed. If present during colonoscopy, the nurse provides client reassurance, support, and technical assistance.

Description of the Procedure: This procedure is performed with inpatients and outpatients and may be performed bedside. The client lies on the left side with legs drawn up to the chest. The colonoscope is inserted through the anus. There may be further movement of the endoscope, i.e., rotation, pulling back, or further insertion, during the procedure. Air may be inserted to allow for closer inspection of the mucosa. When the procedure is complete, the endoscope is withdrawn. Length of time for the procedure depends on what is done during endoscopy and ranges from 10 minutes to 2 hours. The results of visualization are available immediately; results of biopsies or other tests requiring laboratory analysis take longer to obtain.

Evaluating Client Response: Complications following this procedure are rare. The client is observed for unexpected bleeding or sharp pain. Since cramping of the gastrointestinal musculature often occurs, clients frequently complain of pressure or discomfort. Food and medications are resumed. Analgesics are administered as needed. Postprocedure client and family support in dealing with the results is provided.

■ Anoscopy (Proctoscopy, Rigid Sigmoidoscopy, Proctosigmoidoscopy)

Subjective Data: Client complains of change in bowel habits, pain, or fatigue.

Objective Data: Clients may be asymptomatic or may present with altered physical findings and abnormal laboratory blood or stool analyses.

Assessment: Examinations of the anus, rectum, and sigmoid colon are performed with a rigid sigmoidoscope inserted via the anus. Sigmoidoscopy is used to assess clients with suspected ulceration, polyps, or tumors. Sigmoidoscopy is also a routine, periodic screening mechanism for clients over age 50.

Nursing Interventions: Client education includes an explanation of the procedure, bowel preparation, movement of the scope during the procedure, and medications. Scheduling takes into account that this procedure must be performed prior to any barium studies. If biopsy is performed during sigmoidoscopy, follow-up barium studies should be delayed for 3 days. For screening purposes, there may be no bowel preparation. For symptomatic clients, better visualization is achieved when the bowel is empty. The client is on a clear-liquid diet the day prior to examination and is NPO past midnight the night before. To promote emptying of the sigmoid colon prior to the examination, the client receives laxatives, cathartics and/or enemas until the colon is clear. To avoid misleading changes in children, if the mucosa is to be examined, bowel preparation is not performed. Sedatives and/or narcotics are administered prior to and during the procedure to promote client relaxation and reduce muscle spasm. Appropriate precautions, such as raising side rails after giving sedatives or narcotics, are observed. Children usually require less analgesia than adults. If proctosigmoidoscopy is being done at the bedside, the nurse provides client reassurance, support, and technical assistance.

Description of the Procedure: This procedure is performed with inpatients and outpatients and may be performed bedside. The age of the client affects positioning. Infants are placed on the back with knees drawn up and abducted toward the flanks. Adults balance on knees and arms with the knees close to the chest and hands spread on either side of the head. Special tables or pillows are used to help the client maintain this position. For clients who cannot maintain this position, the position described for colonoscopy may be used. The 25–35 cm-long hollow scope is inserted via the anus. Movement of the scope during the procedure may include rotation, pulling back, or further insertion. When the procedure is complete, the scope is withdrawn. Length of time for the procedure depends on what is done during proctosigmoidoscopy and ranges from 10–30 minutes. Results of visualization are available immediately; results of biopsy or other test analyses take longer to obtain.

Evaluating Client Response: Complications following this procedure are rare. The client is monitored for unexpected bleeding or sharp pain. Since cramping of the gastrointestinal musculature frequently occurs, clients may complain of discomfort. Analgesia is administered as appropriate. Food and medications are resumed. Postprocedure client and family support in dealing with the results is provided.

■ Endoscopic Retrograde Cholangiopancreaticography (ERCP, Endoscopic Retrograde Cholangiography, Endoscopic Retrograde Pancreatography)

Subjective Data: Client complains of pain, nausea, or vomiting.

Objective Data: Altered laboratory blood, stool, and urine analyses, and equivocal results from ultrasound, percutaneous transhepatic cholangiography, or CT.

Assessment: ERCP is used to investigate suspected biliary duct pathology. ERCP involves fiberoptic endoscopy and cannulation of the duodenal papilla once the ampulla of Vater is identified. ERCP is the diagnostic method of choice for nonjaundiced clients in whom biliary disease is suspected but is thus far unproven by other testing. ERCP is especially suited for diagnosing pancreatic carcinoma, as it expresses early as ductal abnormalities.

Nursing Interventions: Client education includes an explanation of the procedure, medications, and postprocedure monitoring. The ability of the child to cooperate and the need for additional sedation or restraint is determined. Scheduling takes into account that ERCP is performed prior to any barium studies. If the client has a fever or cholangitis, an antibiotic, i.e., ampicillin 2 g/day 24–48 hours prior to the procedure, may be administered to prevent potential bacteremia induced by endoscopic manipulations. Clients are NPO in advance of ERCP. An IV line may be established for medication administration prior to and during the procedure. A sedative and/or narcotic are administered prior to the procedure. Atropine may also be given to dry secretions. Appropriate precautions, such as raising side rails after giving sedatives or narcotics, are observed. The client is prepared for swallowing the endoscope. Provisions are made for postprocedure monitoring. All jewelry and prostheses are removed. If present during ERCP, the nurse provides client reassurance and technical assistance.

Description of the Procedure: ERCP is performed with inpatients and outpatients. To achieve local anesthesia of the pharynx, either the client gargles with lidocaine or the lidocaine is sprayed on the pharynx. The client is positioned on the left side with the left arm behind the back to make it easier to turn the client prone for cannulation of the duct system. The fiberoptic endoscope is inserted through the mouth. A mouth guard may be inserted to protect client, endoscope, and endoscopist from injury due to biting. The endoscope is advanced via fluoroscopy and the ampulla of Vater identified. A cannula, attached to a contrast-filled syringe, is inserted through the biopsy channel of the endoscope. The duodenal papilla is cannulated and the biliary tract filled with contrast medium. Radiographs are obtained. When completed, the endoscope is withdrawn. ERCP requires approximately 2 hours. The results are available following interpretation.

Evaluating Client Response: Following the procedure, vital signs are monitored and the client is closely observed for dyspnea. Blood in emesis or stool is considered an adverse reaction and the physician is notified. The client is NPO until return of the gag reflex, which is determined by light touch of a tongue blade to the uvula. This may take several hours, depending on the sedation and anesthesia used. Oral intake then begins with ice chips. Close monitoring is maintained to be certain the client swallows with no difficulty. Food and medications are then resumed. Since cramping of the gastrointestinal musculature frequently occurs, clients often complain of discomfort. Analgesia is administered as needed. Post-procedure client and family support in dealing with the results is provided.

BIOPSY

- **Liver Biopsy**
- **Paracentesis**

Biopsy of the GI tract is performed in conjunction with direct visualization. The liver, however, is biopsied by percutaneous aspiration. Samples of ascites fluid are also obtained by percutaneous drainage. A specific consent form is required for these procedures.

Nursing Diagnoses for clients undergoing biopsy include:

- Alteration in comfort related to procedure
- Anxiety related to procedure
- Knowledge deficit related to diagnostic process
- Potential for infection related to procedure
- Potential for injury: bleeding related to procedure

Liver Biopsy

Subjective Data: Client complains of pain or tenderness, nausea, feeling "bloated," increased bleeding, and fatigue.

Objective Data: Altered physical findings including ascites, jaundice, skin changes, altered level of consciousness, gynecomastia, and abnormal results from laboratory and other tests.

Assessment: Percutaneous liver biopsy is performed after other diagnostic procedures have identified a malfunction in the liver. Since the liver is involved in clotting mechanisms, the potential for bleeding is a major concern. Therefore, clotting profiles precede biopsy. Blood typing and cross-matching may also be performed. Some clients receive IM injections of vitamin K prior to a liver biopsy.

Nursing Interventions: Client education includes an explanation of the procedure with emphasis on holding one's breath on command and remaining still. Children may need assistance to remain still. Postprocedure monitoring is explained. The clotting profile, blood typing, and cross-matching are completed as ordered. Vitamin K is administered as ordered. The client may be NPO 6–8 hours prior to the procedure. Baseline vital signs are obtained. If present during the procedure, the nurse provides emotional support and technical assistance.

Description of the Procedure: Liver biopsy is performed with inpatients and on outpatients when sufficient postprocedure monitoring is available. The client is in a supine position, with a small supporting pillow or folded towel under the rib cage on the right side. The client's right hand is placed over the head. The entry site, the sixth intercostal space, is prepared, and local anesthetic is administered. The client is told to take a deep breath and hold the inspiration so that the liver is at its highest point. The aspiration needle is inserted. One ml of saline is inserted to clear the needle of extraneous tissue. The needle is aspirated to obtain liver tissue in the syringe and withdrawn. The procedure is completed in less than 10 minutes. The results are available following laboratory analysis.

Evaluating Client Response: Following the procedure, the client lies on the right side for several hours so the entry site in the liver capsule is compressed against the chest wall. Postprocedure client evaluation includes assessment for potential complications including bleeding at the entry site or in the liver and bile peritonitis. Vital signs are monitored every 15 minutes the first hour, every 30 minutes for the next 2 hours, and prn. The entry site is monitored for bleeding. The client may be on bedrest for up to 24 hours. Food and medications are resumed. Client and family support in dealing with the procedure and results are provided as needed.

■ Paracentesis

Subjective Data: Client complains of pain or tenderness, nausea, vomiting, feeling "bloated," fatigue, or increased bleeding.

Objective Data: Altered physical findings including ascites, jaundice and skin changes, and abnormal laboratory values.

Assessment: Paracentesis, obtaining a sample of ascitic fluid, is performed to confirm the presence of ascites and permit laboratory determination of the components. The fluid is analyzed for protein, amylase, white and red blood cells, cancer cells, fat, specific gravity, or infectious agents. The results are used in ascertaining the reason that the client is accumulating ascites. Only a few milliliters of fluid are removed, thus avoiding the problems associated with large volume fluid shifts within the body. Paracentesis as a treatment mode is considered palliative and is not common.

Nursing Interventions: The procedure is explained to the client. The client voids immediately prior to the procedure in order to decrease bladder size. If present during the procedure, the nurse provides client support and technical assistance.

Description of the Procedure: This procedure is performed with inpatients and outpatients. The client sits upright in a chair with feet on the floor. Baseline vital signs are obtained. The entry site, commonly the midline below the umbilicus, is located and prepared. A trocar, attached by tubing to the collection container, is inserted and several milliliters of ascites drained. The trocar is withdrawn and the entry site covered with a band-aid. This procedure takes less than 10 minutes to complete. The results are available following laboratory analysis.

Evaluating Client Response: Postprocedure evaluation includes frequent monitoring of vital signs. The entry site is observed for potential bleeding or leaking of ascitic fluid. Postprocedure pain is not usual, and if it occurs it should be reported to the physician. Client and family support in dealing with the results is provided.

6

Clients with Impaired Fluid Volume

Impaired fluid volume can arise from different causes. This section focuses on diagnostic procedures for the client with renal and/or urinary tract dysfunction. Other pathophysiologies, however, such as cardiovascular and endocrine malfunction, may also need to be investigated. Many clients with impaired fluid volume experience acid-base and electrolyte imbalances. These problems can be the primary pathophysiology or can be secondary to other disease states. Urinary tract dysfunction frequently causes the client embarrassment. The client's modesty and privacy are protected as much as possible during the diagnostic process and appropriate client support is provided concerning this issue. Nursing diagnoses for clients during the diagnostic process are directed at psychosocial and physiologic needs.

For clients with impaired fluid volume, complete assessment involves several components. A thorough personal history, including customary patterns of fluid intake and voiding, family history, and history of the present illness are mandatory. A detailed recording of the client's subjective complaints is obtained. Physical examination includes inspection, percussion, and palpation of the bladder and kidneys. Other parts of the body, i.e., the skin and dependent areas, are examined for signs of hydration.

The effects of diet, medication, and pathophysiology on urinary output are considered.

For clients with impaired fluid volume, examination of the urine is essential. Urine is assessed in terms of amount, color, clarity, odor, pH, specific gravity, presence of protein, glucose, ketones, red blood cells, white blood cells, casts, crystals, pus, or bacteria. Several urine tests can be performed, with immediate results, wherever the proper equipment is available. Specific gravity is measured by one of the various types of urinometers. Testing for glucose, ketones, protein, blood, and pH may be done individually or together using one of the many products available. It is important to follow specific instructions and note the correct timing sequence and specific drug interactions for each product. Urine samples are refrigerated if not tested immediately to avoid pH changes at room temperature.

Gross microscopic examination will reveal the presence of blood cells, casts, pus, or bacteria. Nevertheless, urine culture and sensitivity, performed on a clean-catch midstream specimen, provides a more detailed report and is the basis for antibiotic therapy. To obtain a clean-catch midstream sample, the client receives a container, antiseptic materials, and instructions. Female clients are told to wipe the skin around the urethra, starting at the front and moving toward the back. Each wipe is used only once. After each side is cleansed, an antiseptic wipe is drawn straight across the urethral opening in the same front to back manner. Male clients are told to retract the foreskin and spread the urinary meatus between thumb and forefinger. The penis is cleansed in a circular motion starting at the meatus and working away. This action is repeated several times with a new antiseptic wipe each time. After cleansing has been completed, the client voids a small amount into the toilet, stops, voids into the collection container, and then finishes voiding into the toilet. The client is instructed not to touch the inside of the collection container or lid, and to replace the lid tightly as soon as possible.

LABORATORY TESTS

Clients with alterations in urinary elimination are likely to undergo repeated laboratory tests. Client cooperation is required for efficient use of time, resources, and money during the diagnostic process.

Nursing Diagnoses for clients undergoing laboratory tests include:

- Anxiety related to procedure
- Knowledge deficit related to diagnostic process

LABORATORY TESTS

Test	Purpose	Normal Values	Nursing Actions
Albumin	Determine		
Urine	presence,	< 5 mg/100 ml	Assist client in
Random	assess renal, cardiac, thyroid status,	No color change	keeping specimen free from vaginal contamination
24-hr	drug toxicity	10–100 mg/24 hr	Collection container must contain preservative or be kept on ice
Aldosterone	Assess en-		
Plasma	docrine status	Fasting, supine: 3–20 ng/100 ml 2hr later, upright: 4–30 ng/100 ml	Varies with sodium diet over prior 2 wk; second sample is taken after breakfast
Urine		2–26 μg/24 hr	Collection container must contain preservative or be kept on ice
Bence-Jones protein Urine, random or 24-hr	Assess renal function, oncologic status	Negative	Test specimen as soon as possible; keep container on ice
Blood urea nitrogen (BUN) Serum	Assess renal function, hydration status	Adult: 10–20 mg/100 ml Child: 8–18 mg/100 ml Newborn: 5–15 mg/100 ml	

(Continued)

LABORATORY TESTS (cont.)

Test	Purpose	Normal Values	Nursing Actions
Electrolytes:			
Calcium (Ca^{++}) Serum	Assess renal, neuromuscular, bone status; parathyroid, thyroid function	Adult: 8.5–10.5 mg/100 ml Child: 8–11 mg/100 ml	
Urine		50–150 mg/24 hr varies with diet	
Chloride (CL^{-}) Serum	Assess renal status, acid-base balance, Addison's disease	Adult: 95–105 mEq/L Child: 96–105 mEq/L	
Urine		110–254 mEq/24 hr varies with diet	Collection container must contain preservative or be kept on ice
Sweat	Assess for cystic fibrosis	10–35 mEq/L	
Magnesium (Mg^{++}) Serum	Assess renal, metabolic, neuromuscular, status	Adult: 1.4–2.3 mEq/L Child: 1.4–1.9 mEq/L	
Urine		6–8.5 mEq/L	
Phosphorus (PO_4) Serum	Assess renal, parathyroid function, bone status	Adult: 2.5–4.5 mg/100 ml Child: 3.6–6.5 mg/100 ml	
Urine		900–1300 mg/24 hr	
Potassium Serum	Assess renal status, endocrine, cardiac function, acid-base balance	Adult and child: 3.5–5.0 mEq/L Newborn: 5.0–7.7 mEq/L	
Urine		Adult and child: 25–120 mEq/24 hr varies with diet	

Test	Purpose	Normal Values	Nursing Actions
Sodium (Na^+)	Assess renal status, endocrine function, acid-base balance		
Serum		134–145 mEq/L	
Urine		40–220 mEq/24 hr varies with diet	
Sweat	Assess cystic fibrosis	Adult: 0–90 μmole/L Child: 0–50 μmole/L Infant: 0–40 μmole/L	
Creatinine	Assess renal urinary tract function, bone status, muscular dystrophy		
Serum		Adult: 0.7–1.4 mg/100 ml Child: 0.3–0.8 mg/100 ml Infant: 0.2/0.5 mg/100 ml	
Urine		Male: 1.0–2.0 g/24 hr Female: 0.8–1.8 g/24 hr	Collection container must contain preservative or be kept on ice
Creatinine clearance Urine and serum		Adult: 75–125 ml/min Child: 95–150 ml/min	24-hr collection container must contain preservative or be kept on ice; A serum level is drawn to coincide with the last urine sample collected
Fishberg concentration test Urine	Assess ability of the kidneys to conserve fluid; differentiate diabetes insipidous and psychogenic polydipsia	Adult: Urine volume: <300 ml Specific gravity: >1.024 Osmolality: >850 mOsm	Clients are NPO for 12 hr overnight; 3 hourly specimens are collected; No intake is allowed during the test

(Continued)

LABORATORY TESTS (cont.)

Test	Purpose	Normal Values	Nursing Actions
Furosemide	Determine level,	Toxic: >25 μg/ml	
Osmolality Serum	Assess renal, endocrine function	285–308 mOsm/kg H_2O	
Urine		250–1200 mOsm/kg H_2O	
Serum/urine ratio		>1 : <3.0	
Uric acid Serum	Assess renal function, gout, lead poisoning	Female: 2.2–7.7 mg/100 ml Male: 3.9–9.0 mg/100 ml	
Urinalysis	Screening tool; assess renal, endocrine status, infection	Color, Turbidity: clear Negative for: glucose, ketones, blood, bile, protein, bilirubin, crystals, RBC, WBC Casts: not waxy; few hyaline, epithelial, or granular	Urine sample must be fresh for accurate results
Specific gravity		1.010–1.025	
pH		5.0–7.5	
Urine culture	Determine presence of pathogens	Negative, or <10,000 organisms/ml	Use clean-catch procedure to obtain uncontaminated specimen
Vanillylmandelic acid (VMA, catecholamines, 3-methoxy-4 methoxy acid) Urine	Determine level, assess adrenal function	VMA: 0–12 mg/24 hr Epinephrine: 100–230/24 hr Metanephrine: 24–96/24 hr Normetanephrine: 12–288/24 hr	Determine client cooperation with specific prespecimen collection VMA diet Collection container must contain preservative or be kept on ice

Please note, normal values are guidelines. Please check with the laboratory performing the test for absolute values.

ULTRASONOGRAPHY

Ultrasound is used to examine clients with impaired fluid volume because it is accurate, does not expose the client to ionizing radiation or iodinated contrast medium, and because renal status does not affect testing. A specific consent form may be required.

Nursing Diagnoses for clients undergoing ultrasound include:

- Anxiety related to procedure
- Alteration in comfort, bladder distension related to procedure
- Knowledge deficit related to diagnostic process

Subjective Data: Client complains of changes in micturition, dysuria, or tenderness.

Objective Data: Hematuria, symptoms of electrolyte imbalance such as edema, nausea, vomiting, or fatigue, proteinuria, or other abnormal laboratory findings.

Assessment: Renal ultrasonography is the diagnostic method of choice for clients with high levels of azotemia, elevated BUN, rising creatinine levels, low urine output, or concomitant other pathophysiologies. Ultrasound can determine whether the kidney is blocked. It is used for clients with clinical evidence of hydronephrosis, adult polycystic disease, infantile polycystic disease, medullary cystic disease, renal cortex disease, renal lesions, neoplasms, or kidney transplants. Ultrasound is used to locate abscesses within infected kidneys. Based on individual need, ultrasound examination of the kidney includes varied client positions for longitudinal and/or transverse imaging using gray-scale and/or real-time ultrasound techniques.

The bladder is usually examined transabdominally. More rarely, sonoendoscopy, insertion of the transducer into the bladder, via the urethra, or a transrectal sonoendoscopic probe, for prostate evaluation, may be used. The bladder is examined for volume, retention, calculi, diverticuli, or tumor. A full, distended bladder promotes visualization by displacing the bowel from the pelvis and eliminating interference from bowel gas. The ureters do not lend themselves to ultrasonic evaluation.

Nursing Interventions: Client education includes an explanation of the procedure including positioning, remaining still, and feeling some pressure during the procedure. Children may need assistance with positioning.

Placement of the transducer is explained. For optimal ultrasonic visualization of the bladder, but not kidney, the client's bladder must be full and distended. The nurse provides instructions regarding drinking approximately 1 liter of fluid prior to the procedure and access to a bathroom following completion of the study.

Description of the Procedure: This procedure is performed with inpatients and outpatients. The client goes to the ultrasound area and reclines. Position varies for renal ultrasonography depending on the view needed. Bladder ultrasonography is performed with the client supine. For sonoendoscopy, the client is in the lithotomy position, whereas transrectal sonography is performed with the client in the lithotomy, left-lateral-decubitus, or knee–chest position. Privacy is assured. Conductive oil or gel is applied to the abdomen for optimal contact between transducer and skin. The transducer is moved across the skin according to the type of ultrasound examination being performed. Ultrasound examinations take approximately 30 minutes to complete. The results are available following interpretation.

Evaluating Client Response: Client and family support in dealing with the results is provided as needed.

MAGNETIC RESONANCE IMAGING (NUCLEAR MAGNETIC IMAGING, MR, NMR)

MR is being used for clients with impaired fluid volume. Bone does not interfere and bowel gas can actually enhance the study. MR has shown potential for use in assessing renal and bladder disease. A specific consent form may be required.

Nursing Diagnoses for clients undergoing MR include:

- Anxiety related to procedure
- Knowledge deficit related to diagnostic procedure

Subjective Data: Client complains of pain or changes in voiding.

Objective Data: Edema, nausea, fatigue, and altered physical or laboratory findings.

Assessment: MR can demonstrate bladder tumors, metastatic spread to surrounding organs, and the level of pelvic obstruction. MR can identify bladder outlet obstruction or carcinoma of the bladder wall and is used to differentiate benign prostatic hypertrophy from prostatic cancer. MR is contraindicated in clients with aneurysm clips anywhere in the body, or with pacemakers because of the effect of the magnetic field.

Nursing Interventions: Client education includes the need to remain still during imaging. The ability of the child to cooperate is determined. Sedation and restraints are usually required for infants and young children. Clients are prepared for the imposing size of the MR scanner, and the noninvasive nature of the procedure is emphasized. A client health history specific to past insertion of aneurysm clips or a pacemaker is obtained. The client changes into a hospital gown, removes all jewelry and prostheses, and voids prior to the procedure.

Description of the Procedure: MR is performed with inpatients and outpatients. The client goes to the MR room and lies supine within the body scanner during the scanning procedure. Completion time depends upon image quality and may take up to 1 hour. Results are available after interpretation.

Evaluating Client Response: Postprocedure client and family support in dealing with the results is provided as needed.

UROPYNAMIC MEASUREMENTS

- **Uroflowmetry**
- **Urethral Pressure Profile**
- **Cystometrography**

Urodynamic measurements provide quantitative data regarding bladder function. Client cooperation is essential and comprehensive client preparation is mandated. A specific consent form may be required for these procedures.

Nursing Diagnoses for clients undergoing urodynamic measurement include:

- ▶ Alteration in comfort related to procedure
- ▶ Anxiety related to procedure
- ▶ Knowledge deficit related to diagnostic process

■ Uroflowmetry

Subjective Data: Client complains of pain, frequency, and difficulty in voiding.

Objective Data: History of repeated urinary tract infection or bladder dysfunction as evidenced by retention, incontinence, or encopresis.

Assessment: Uroflowmetry is a simple, noninvasive test that measures and records urine flow through the urethra. The client voids as usual into a specially constructed commode. The urine flow is recorded in ml/sec.

Nursing Interventions: Client education includes an explanation of the procedure. The ability of the child to participate is determined. Children must be able to cooperate by not having a bowel movement during the procedure. Older children and adults may need assistance in dealing with concerns about modesty, privacy, and urinating in front of others. The client is encouraged to drink so as to be well-hydrated prior to the procedure. If present during this procedure, the nurse provides client support and technical assistance.

Description of the Procedure: This procedure is performed with inpatients and outpatients. In the urology laboratory, the client sits on the commode and voids as usual. Urine flow is measured and recorded. Uroflowmetry is complete in less than 30 minutes. The results may be available immediately or following later interpretation.

Evaluating Client Response: Postprocedure client and family support in dealing with the result is provided.

■ Urethral Pressure Profile

Subjective Data: Client complains of pain, frequency, and difficulty in voiding.

Objective Data: History of repeated urinary tract infection or bladder dysfunction as evidenced by retention, incontinence, or encopresis.

Assessment: Urethral pressure profile provides a graphic recording of urethral pressure. Readings are obtained along the entire course of the urethra from the bladder neck to the meatus. Urethral pressure profiles are not performed on clients with acute urinary tract infections.

Nursing Interventions: Client education includes an explanation of the procedure. Children may need assistance in lying still. The client is supported while dealing with concerns about modesty. If present during the procedure, the nurse provides client support and technical assistance.

Description of the Procedure: This procedure is performed with inpatients and outpatients. The client wears a hospital gown and goes to the urology laboratory. The client is asked to void. A thin straight catheter is inserted under sterile technique into the bladder. As sterile irrigating fluid or carbon dioxide is inserted into the urethra, the catheter is slowly withdrawn and pressure in the urethra measured and recorded. Measurements may be obtained at different levels of bladder fullness. Urethral pressure profiles are complete in less than 30 minutes. The results may be available immediately or following later interpretation.

Evaluating Client Response: Intake and output are monitored. The time, color, and amount of the first voiding are recorded. Mild hematuria is to be expected, but persistent hematuria or fever are reported to the physician. Client complaints of burning on urination or discomfort are expected. Warm baths and/or analgesia are provided as needed. Client and family support in dealing with the results is provided.

■ Cystometrography

Subjective Data: Client complains of pain, frequency, and difficulty in voiding.

Objective Data: History of repeated urinary tract infection or bladder dysfunction as evidenced by retention, incontinence, or encopresis.

Assessment: Cystometrography provides a graphic recording of pressure changes during bladder function. Bladder capacity, efficiency of the detrusor muscle, intravesical pressure, and sensory reaction to hot and cold stimuli are measured in clients with evidence of neurogenic bladder or loss of bladder muscle tone. Cystometrography is not performed on clients with acute urinary tract infections.

Nursing Interventions: Client education includes a detailed description of the procedure and the possibility of several repetitions. The ability of the child to participate is determined. Children must be able to cooperate by not having a bowel movement during the procedure. In younger children, intrabladder pressures can be measured leaving the catheter in place and using carbon dioxide to inflate the bladder. Older children and adults need assistance in dealing with concerns about modesty, privacy, and urinating in front of others. If present during this procedure, the nurse provides client support and technical assistance.

Description of the Procedure: This procedure is performed with inpatients and outpatients. The client wears a hospital gown and goes to the urology laboratory. The client is asked to void. Notation is made regarding how long it takes the client to begin voiding and the force and continuity of the urinary stream. The client assumes the lithotomy position. Under sterile technique, a catheter is inserted into the bladder. Residual volume is measured. The catheter is connected to a manometer and sterile water is inserted into the bladder at a constant rate. In some instances, carbon dioxide is used instead of water for bladder inflation. The client is asked to report first feeling the urge to void and feeling a full bladder. These and other pressures are recorded. The catheter is removed. Bladder sensory response may be assessed by the insertion of cold and then warm water. Stress incontinence may be assessed by having the client cough when the bladder is full. The client voids and the same data as above is noted. This series of voiding, catheter insertion, measuring for retention, bladder filling, recording pressures, and voiding may be repeated several times. Cystometrography is completed in approximately 1–2 hours. The results may be available immediately or following later interpretation.

Evaluating Client Response: Intake and output are monitored. The time, color, and amount of the first voiding are recorded. Mild hematuria is to be expected, but persistent hematuria or fever are reported to the physician. Client complaints of burning on urination or discomfort are expected. Warm baths and/or analgesia are provided as needed. Client and family support in dealing with the results is provided.

SCINTIGRAPHY

- **Kidney Scan**
- **Renogram**
- **Diuretic Radionuclide Urogram**
- **Radionuclide Cystogram**

Scintigraphy is used to assess size, location, and shape of the kidneys. It can also assess pathophysiology and quantitate diuretic function. A specific consent form may be required for these procedures.

Nursing Diagnoses for clients undergoing scintigraphy include:

- Anxiety related to procedure
- Knowledge deficit related to diagnostic process

■ Kidney Scan (Renal Scan and Perfusion Study)

Subjective Data: Client complains of pain, malaise, or changes in voiding.

Objective Data: Altered physical findings including hypertension and abnormal laboratory analysis of blood and/or urine.

Assessment: Renal scans provide data on kidney size, shape, location, perfusion, and function for clients with impaired fluid volume. Suspected tubular disease, urinary obstruction, pyelonephritis, cyst, or tumor can be examined. Failure of the kidneys to visualize is associated with a poor client prognosis. IV injection of the radioisotope precedes scanning. Scintigraphy is contraindicated during pregnancy and lactation.

Nursing Interventions: Client education includes an explanation of the procedure and positioning. Children may need help staying still. The IV injections, repeated imagings, and time framework are discussed. A client history specific for pregnancy, allergy to iodine, and previous reaction to contrast medium is obtained. Potential cross-interference is reduced by allowing 24–48 hours between different nuclear medicine studies. Retained barium from any previous examination will easily destroy scintigraphic results. All jewelry is removed.

Description of the Procedure: This procedure is performed with inpatients and outpatients. The client either sits or stands and receives an IV injection in order to determine positioning for client and cameras during this study. A second IV injection containing the radioisotope is administered and imaging starts immediately in order to demonstrate blood flow. Approximately 30 minutes later, images of the kidneys are obtained. Radiographs may also be obtained. This procedure is completed in 1–2 hours. Follow-up imaging may be required over several hours. The results are available following interpretation.

Evaluating Client Response: Postprocedure support for client and family in dealing with the results is provided.

■ Renogram (Renocystogram)

Subjective Data: Client complains of pain, malaise, or changes in voiding.

Objective Data: Altered physical findings including hypertension and abnormal laboratory analysis of blood and/or urine.

Assessment: Renograms provide data regarding renal perfusion and function. Two gamma cameras are used for imaging following IV injection of the radionuclide. Excretion time activity curves quantify transit of the radionuclide through the kidney. Normally, blood flow through the two kidneys is equal, and 50% of the radioisotope is excreted in 10 minutes. Scintigraphy is contraindicated during pregnancy and lactation.

Nursing Interventions: The procedure is explained to the client. Children may need help staying still. A client history specific for pregnancy, allergy to iodine, and previous reaction to contrast medium is obtained. Potential cross-interference is reduced by allowing 24–48 hours between different nuclear medicine studies. Retained barium from any previous examination will easily destroy scintigraphic results. The client is well-hydrated. All jewelry is removed.

Description of the Procedure: This procedure is performed with inpatients and outpatients. In the nuclear medicine department, the client assumes a sitting or supine position. An IV injection may be given to help establish client and camera position for this study. A Gamma camera is positioned over each kidney. The radionuclide is then injected intravenously as scanning begins simultaneously. This procedure is completed in approximately 1 hour. The results are available following interpretation.

Evaluating Client Response: Postprocedure support for client and family in dealing with the results is provided.

■ Diuretic Radionuclide Urogram

Subjective Data: Client complains of pain or changes in voiding.

Objective Data: Altered physical findings and abnormal laboratory analysis of blood and/or urine.

Assessment: This study is used to differentiate obstructed and non-obstructed dilated pelvocalyceal states. Time activity curves are obtained from the upper and lower portions of the ureter or bladder both before and after IV administration of furosemide. If activity in the upper ureter falls after diuresis, the system is not obstructed. Scintigraphy is contraindicated during pregnancy and lactation.

Nursing Interventions: Client education includes an explanation of the procedure and positioning. Children may need help staying still. The diuretic effects of furosemide are explained. A client history specific for pregnancy, allergy to iodine, and previous reaction to contrast medium is obtained. Potential cross-interference is reduced by allowing 24–48 hours between different nuclear medicine studies. Retained barium from any previous examination will easily destroy scintigraphic results. All jewelry is removed.

Description of the Procedure: This procedure is performed with inpatients and outpatients. The client goes to the nuclear medicine department. Since the client will receive several IV injections, a heparin lock or continuous IV infusion is initiated. The client assumes a sitting or standing position. A Gamma camera is positioned over each kidney. The radionuclide is injected intravenously and scanning begun simultaneously. After the radioisotope has cleared the kidneys, furosemide is administered intravenously. Additional radionuclide is then injected and imaging repeated. This procedure is completed in approximately 2–3 hours. Before and after diuretic renal excretion times are calculated and compared. The results are available following interpretation.

Evaluating Client Response: Postprocedure support for client and family in dealing with the results is provided.

■ Radionuclide Cystogram

Subjective Data: Client complains of discomfort or difficulty in voiding.

Objective Data: Altered physical findings and abnormal laboratory analysis of blood and/or urine.

Assessment: Radionuclide cystography is used to assess vesicoureteral reflux. Imaging takes place following insertion of the radionuclide via catheter, following the client's urge to void and following removal of the catheter and voiding. Scintigraphy is contraindicated during pregnancy and lactation.

Nursing Interventions: Client education includes an explanation of the procedure. The ability of the child to participate is determined. The client is made aware that the procedure may take $5\frac{1}{2}$ hours. A client history specific for pregnancy, allergy to iodine, and previous reaction to contrast medium is obtained. Potential cross-interference is reduced by allowing 24–48 hours between different nuclear medicine studies. Retained barium from any previous examination easily destroys scintigraphic results. All jewelry and prostheses are removed.

Description of the Procedure: This procedure is performed with inpatients and outpatients. In the nuclear medicine department, the client may be asked to drink some fluid immediately prior to the procedure. The client assumes the lithotomy position and a catheter is inserted into the bladder. The radionuclide is instilled and the catheter clamped. Imaging is started immediately. When the client expresses the urge to void, scintigraphs are obtained as the client strains against the catheter. The clamp is removed and further scintigraphs obtained as the client voids through the catheter. The catheter is removed and additional scintigraphs may be obtained over several hours. This procedure takes 1 hour plus additional scintigraphy as desired. The results are available following interpretation.

Evaluating Client Response: Postprocedure support for client and family in dealing with the results is provided.

RADIOLOGY (KIDNEY URETER BLADDER FILMS, KUB)

For clients with impaired fluid volume, x-rays demonstrate size, shape, and position of the kidneys as well as some pathologies. A specific consent form may be required.

Nursing Diagnoses for clients undergoing radiographs include:

- Anxiety related to procedure
- Knowledge deficit related to diagnostic process

Subjective Data: Client complains of pelvic or abdominal pain or changes in voiding.

Objective Data: Altered physical findings or laboratory data.

Assessment: Calcification in the kidneys, hydronephrosis, displacement by surrounding tissue, and urinary tract cysts or tumors are evident on x-rays. More than 90% of renal calculi are identified on abdominal x-ray. KUB radiographs are used in clients with suspected emphysematous pyelonephritis to demonstrate gas outside the bowel lumen.

Nursing Interventions: The procedure is explained to the client. Scheduling takes into account that abdominal and KUB radiographs may be ineffective when they follow barium or other ingested or rectally inserted contrast media exams. KUB films are contraindicated during pregnancy. The client wears a hospital gown and removes all jewelry and prostheses.

Description of the Procedure: This procedure is done with inpatients and outpatients. The client stands and is positioned relative to the camera. The client may be asked to inspire and hold a deep breath. This test takes less than 5 minutes. The results are available following interpretation.

Evaluating Client Response: Postprocedure support for client and family is provided as they deal with the need for further diagnostic testing.

COMPUTED TOMOGRAPHY (CT, COMPUTERIZED AXIAL TOMOGRAPHY, CAT SCAN, EMI)

Computed tomography is used to assess clients with impaired fluid volume. Kidneys and bladder may be examined for obstruction, calculi, or mass. CT study may follow equivocal sonography. CT scanning involves several views, but since scatter radiation is limited, the effects are not additive and each section receives only its own exposure. Renal and bladder CT are contraindicated during pregnancy. A specific consent form may be required.

Nursing Diagnoses for clients undergoing CT include:

- Anxiety related to procedure
- Knowledge deficit related to diagnostic process
- Potential for injury: allergic reaction related to procedure

Subjective Data: Client complains of changes in voiding or pain.

Objective Data: The client demonstrates symptoms of electrolyte imbalance such as edema, hematuria, proteinuria, or other abnormal laboratory data and equivocal findings on ultrasound.

Assessment: Renal CT scans are performed with and without contrast media. Noncontrast scans are highly reliable for detecting small calculi. Contrast-enhanced CT provides a definitive description of renal abscesses and is effective in staging renal carcinoma. CT is used to delineate retroperitoneal abnormalities such as lymphadenopathy responsible for hydronephrosis. Contrast medium may be injected through the pedal vein to opacify the vena cava if involvement of that vein is suspected.

Bladder CT is used to locate masses within the bladder and those externally obstructing urine flow. For an in-depth bladder analysis, CT is performed with IV iodinated contrast medium. Blocking agents, e.g., Lugol's solution, are administered. Double contrast studies involve contrast medium and residual urine, whereas triple contrast studies also add air to the bladder. To delineate the perivesical space, the bowel lumen is opacified by the client's oral ingestion of contrast medium and may be further enhanced by rectal administration of contrast medium.

Nursing Interventions: Client education prior to CT scanning includes an explanation of the procedure and the need to remain still during imaging. The ability of the child to cooperate by lying still and the need for sedation or restraint is determined. The client is prepared for administration of the contrast medium. The imposing size of the CT scanner is explained and the noninvasive nature of the procedure is emphasized. A history specific as to pregnancy is obtained, and for contrast-enhanced scans, allergy to iodine, or previous reaction to contrast medium is also determined. Clients are frequently NPO 2–4 hours prior to CT scans, especially for contrast-enhanced scans. Clear liquids may be permitted. The client changes into a hospital gown, removes all jewelry and prostheses, voids and goes to the CT room.

Description of the Procedure: CT is performed with inpatients and outpatients. Administration of contrast medium may precede CT scanning by 1 hour. The contrast medium for renal CT scanning is administered intravenously. For perivesical space opacification, the client drinks 500 ml of water-soluble oral contrast material 1 hour prior to the exam. Water-soluble contrast material, 250–300 ml, is then administered rectally just prior to the study. For bladder study, contrast medium is administered intravenously. Air is inserted if needed. The client is supine within the body scanner. Suspended respiration is not required for bladder CT unless there is an unusually long scan time. This procedure is completed in approximately 30 minutes. Results are available after interpretation.

Evaluating Client Response: Following the procedure, food and medications are resumed. Fluid intake is encouraged to assist in eliminating the contrast medium. Postprocedure client and family support in dealing with the results is provided.

CONTRAST STUDIES

- **Intravenous Urogram**
- **Infusion Drip Pyelogram**
- **Retrograde Pyelogram**
- **Cystourethrogram**
- **Retrograde Urethrogram**
- **Digital Subtraction Angiography**
- **Renal Angiography**

Contrast studies are a major diagnostic tool for clients with impaired fluid volume. Visualization is achieved by IV injection of contrast medium or by insertion of radiopaque material into the desired area. A specific consent form is required for these procedures.

Nursing Diagnoses for clients undergoing contrast studies include:

- Alteration in comfort related to procedure
- Anxiety related to procedure
- Knowledge deficit related to diagnostic process
- Potential for injury: allergic reaction related to procedure

Intravenous Urogram (IVU, Intravenous Pyelography, IVP, Excretory Urogram)

Subjective Data: Client complains of pain, frequency, and difficulty voiding.

Objective Data: Altered physical findings including hypertension, repeated urinary problems, and abnormal laboratory analyses of blood and/or urine.

Assessment: IVU is performed early in the diagnostic process. Contrast medium is injected intravenously and concentrates in the urine, thus promoting visualization of the kidneys, ureters, and bladder. IVU provides anatomic and functional information about obstructions, bladder abnormalities, glomerulonephritis, renal hematoma, and congenital abnormalities. IVU is the standard imaging procedure for identifying renal masses and the simplest method for locating calcifications within the collecting system or ureters. IVU is contraindicated during pregnancy.

Nursing Interventions: Client education includes an explanation of the procedure. The client is prepared for potential flushed and/or nauseous sensations during contrast medium injection. Children may require additional assistance during the test. The client is instructed regarding post-procedure fluid intake and is told that urine may be discolored from the contrast medium. If performed on an outpatient basis, the client must be willing and able to comply with the preprocedure regimen. A client history specific for pregnancy, allergy to iodine, and previous reaction to contrast medium is obtained. Barium studies cannot precede IVU. Protocol for bowel preparation varies by institution, but commonly includes a laxative the night before the exam to eliminate feces and intestinal gas. The client is NPO for 12 hours prior to the exam unless dehydration is of concern. Clear liquids may be permitted. Infants are only slightly dehydrated prior to the procedure. The client wears a hospital gown and removes all jewelry and prostheses.

Description of the Procedure: IVU is performed with inpatients and outpatients. The client lies supine on the radiology table. An IV line is inserted and the contrast medium injected. Serial timed radiographs are obtained. An IVP is completed in approximately 1 hour. Preliminary results may be available immediately, but definitive diagnosis follows interpretation.

Evaluating Client Response: Postprocedure client evaluation includes assessment for contrast medium reaction. Vital signs are monitored. Fluid intake is encouraged to promote excretion of the contrast medium. Food and medications are resumed. Client and family support in dealing with the results and the need for any further testing is provided.

■ Infusion Drip Pyelogram (Nephrotomogram)

Subjective Data: Client complains of pain, frequency, and difficulty voiding.

Objective Data: Altered physical findings and equivocal results from other laboratory and diagnostic tests.

Assessment: Infusion drip pyelography is performed when other urographic techniques have failed to adequately demonstrate the drainage structure satisfactorily or when tomograms are needed. Large quantities of dilute contrast medium are injected intravenously and provide for opacification of the renal parenchyma and complete filling of the urinary tract. Serial radiographs and nephrotomograms (body section radiographs) are obtained. This procedure is contraindicated during pregnancy.

Nursing Interventions: Client education includes an explanation of the procedure. Children may require additional assistance during the test. The client is told that the contrast medium may cause the urine to be discolored after the procedure. A client history specific for pregnancy, allergy to iodine, and previous reaction to contrast medium is obtained. Barium studies cannot precede this test. Clients may receive a laxative the night before the exam to eliminate feces and intestinal gas. Because the contrast medium is so dilute, nausea upon injection is uncommon and these clients are not usually NPO prior to the exam. The client wears a hospital gown and removes all jewelry and prostheses.

Description of the Procedure: This procedure is performed on inpatients and outpatients. The client lies supine on the radiology table. An IV line is inserted and the dilute contrast medium injected slowly during the procedure. Serial timed radiographs and nephrotomograms are obtained. Infusion drip pyelography is completed in 1–2 hours. Preliminary results may be available immediately, but definitive diagnosis follows interpretation.

Evaluating Client Response: Postprocedure client evaluation includes assessment for contrast medium reaction. Vital signs are monitored. Fluid intake is encouraged to promote excretion of the contrast medium. Client and family support in dealing with the results is provided.

■ Retrograde Pyelogram and Cystogram

Subjective Data: Client complains of pain, frequency, and difficulty voiding.

Objective Data: Altered physical findings including hypertension, repeated urinary problems, and abnormal laboratory analyses of blood and/or urine.

Assessment: These two procedures (retrograde pyelogram and cystogram) are performed using similar technique. Retrograde pyelography provides data on the anatomical structure of the kidneys and is performed if IVU has resulted in inadequate visualization of the collecting system or if lesions of the ureters are suspected. The radiopaque contrast medium is inserted via cystoscopy. Cystography is used to examine the bladder wall, detect calculi in the bladder, and evaluate any vesicouretal reflux, i.e., backwards flow from the bladder into the ureters. Radiopaque contrast medium is injected through a catheter inserted into the bladder. Although the contrast medium is not injected intravenously, a small amount may be absorbed across the urinary mucosa and caution is maintained for clients with a history of prior allergic reaction. These procedures are contraindicated during pregnancy.

Nursing Interventions: Client education includes an explanation of cystoscopy, the radiologic procedure, and the importance of client cooperation. Children may require additional assistance during the test. Clients receive instructions regarding a high fluid intake following the procedure and the potential for urine discoloration from the contrast medium. A client history specific for pregnancy, allergy to iodine, and previous reaction to contrast medium is obtained. Barium studies cannot precede these tests. Clients are NPO past midnight prior to this procedure and receive bowel preparation, commonly a laxative the night before the exam, to eliminate feces and intestinal gas. Preprocedure sedation may be administered. The client wears a hospital gown and removes all jewelry and prostheses.

Description of the Procedure: These procedures are performed with inpatients and outpatients. The client has an IV line inserted for sedative administration. Some clients may receive general anesthesia. The client assumes the lithotomy position on the radiology table. Local anesthetic is applied to the urethra. The cystoscope is inserted and a catheter threaded through the cystoscope and, via fluoroscopy, up the ureters into the renal pelvis. Radiopaque contrast medium is inserted. Serial radiographs are obtained. Retrograde pyelography is completed in approximately 2 hours. Preliminary results may be available immediately, but definitive diagnosis follows interpretation.

Evaluating Client Response: Postprocedure client evaluation includes assessment for contrast medium reaction, bleeding, or pain. Vital signs are monitored. Food and medications are resumed. Fluid intake is encouraged to promote excretion of the contrast medium. If the client received general anesthesia, the associated nursing responsibilities are implemented. Client and family support in dealing with the results is provided.

■ Cystourethrogram (Voiding Cystourethrogram, Micturating Cystourethrogram, MCU)

Subjective Data: Client complains of pain and difficulty voiding.

Objective Data: Altered physical findings including repeated urinary problems and abnormal laboratory analyses of blood and/or urine.

Assessment: Cystourethrography is used to assess lower urinary tract obstructions, strictures, lacerations, trauma, congenital abnormality, or bladder neck spasms in paraplegic clients. Suspected ureteric reflux, such as occurs in children with repeated urinary tract infections, may be examined. A catheter is inserted into the bladder, which visualizes following instillation of the radiopaque medium. For a voiding study, contrast medium is instilled in the bladder, the catheter is removed, and rapid serial radiographs obtained as the client voids. This study is contraindicated in the presence of acute urinary tract infection and during pregnancy. Since small amounts of contrast medium may be absorbed across the urinary tract mucosa, caution is maintained for clients with prior allergic reaction.

Nursing Interventions: Client education includes an explanation of the procedure, including catheter insertion, and the importance of client cooperation. Children may need additional assistance, restraints, or sedation during this procedure. A client history specific for pregnancy, allergy to iodine, and previous reaction to contrast medium is obtained. Barium studies cannot precede this test. Clients are permitted no food for 12 hours prior to the test but are allowed clear liquids to drink. The client wears a hospital gown and removes all jewelry and prostheses.

Description of the Procedure: This procedure is performed on inpatients and outpatients. The client assumes the lithotomy position on the radiology table. Local anesthesia may be applied to the urethra. The catheter is inserted into the bladder. Contrast medium is inserted and serial radiographs are obtained. For a voiding study, the catheter is removed and radiographs obtained as the client voids. Clients may be asked to change positions for different views. MCU is completed in 1–2 hours. Preliminary results may be available immediately, but definitive diagnosis follows interpretation.

Evaluating Client Response: Postprocedure client evaluation includes assessment for allergic reaction. Client and family support in dealing with the results is provided.

■ Retrograde Urethrogram

Subjective Data: Client complains of pain and difficulty voiding.

Objective Data: Altered physical findings including repeated urinary problems and abnormal laboratory analyses of blood and/or urine.

Assessment: Retrograde urethrography is used in male clients to assess the site, severity, and number of urethral strictures. It is performed by retrograde injection of contrast medium into the external urethral meatus. This procedure is contraindicated within 7 days of urethral instrumentation or in the presence of acute urethral infection. Since small amounts of contrast medium may be absorbed across the urinary tract mucosa, caution is maintained for clients with prior allergic reaction.

Nursing Interventions: Client education includes an explanation of the procedure, including catheter insertion, and the importance of client cooperation. Children may need additional assistance during this test. A client history specific for allergy to iodine and previous reaction to contrast medium is obtained. Barium studies cannot precede this procedure. The client wears a hospital gown and removes all jewelry and prostheses.

Description of the Procedure: This procedure is performed with inpatients and outpatients. The client reclines on the radiology table. A catheter is inserted into the external urinary meatus and contrast medium is inserted. Radiographs are obtained. Retrograde urethrography is completed in approximately 1 hour. Preliminary results may be available immediately, but definitive diagnosis follows interpretation.

Evaluating Client Response: Postprocedure client evaluation includes assessment for contrast medium reaction. Client and family support in dealing with the results is provided.

■ Digital Subtraction Angiography (DSA)

Subjective Data: Client complains of headaches or throbbing.

Objective Data: Hypertension of undetermined origin.

Assessment: This procedure uses an image enhancement system, known as "mask mode subtraction," to amplify low concentration intravascular iodine signals to obtain data about arterial blood flow. Intravenous DSA is used as the initial radiologic procedure for clients with hypertension of suspected renovascular etiology. IV DSA is also used to assess potential kidney donors and kidney transplant recipients with hypertension. This procedure is contraindicated during pregnancy.

Nursing Interventions: Client education includes an explanation of the procedure and the need to remain still. The ability of the client to lie perfectly still has a major impact on the success of this procedure. DSA may not be suitable for children, depending on their ability to cooperate. A client history specific for pregnancy, allergy to iodine, or previous reaction to contrast medium is obtained. Adequacy of kidney function is determined as the client receives 150–250 ml of contrast medium solution over 30–60 minutes. Clients may be NPO for 2 hours before the procedure. Premedication is not usually necessary. The client wears a hospital gown, removes all jewelry and prostheses, and voids prior to the procedure.

Description of the Procedure: IV DSA is performed with inpatients and outpatients. The client goes to the radiology department, reclines and is positioned relative to the fluoroscopic camera. If indicated, the client's ECG is monitored. The mask is recorded and stored by computer. The entry site is prepared. The contrast medium is administered intravenously. The second image is obtained. Movement makes the mask unsatisfactory. If this occurs, another mask can be obtained after the contrast media has left the region. DSA is completed in less than 1 hour. Results are available following interpretation.

Evaluating Client Response: Following IV DSA, the insertion site is checked for signs of bleeding. Medication and food are resumed and pain medications are administered as needed. Clients are encouraged to increase fluid intake to approximately 2 liters to promote excretion of the contrast medium. Outpatients are instructed to check for postprocedure bleeding and return immediately if any bleeding is noted. Outpatients should not drive home. Client and family support is provided.

■ Renal Angiography

Subjective Data: Client complains of pain or malaise.

Objective Data: Altered physical findings including hypertension and other abnormal diagnostic data and laboratory tests.

Assessment: Clients with impaired fluid volume may undergo angiography of the kidney. Renal angiography assesses renal circulation and stenosis, abnormal vasculature or mass. A catheter is threaded via fluoroscopy to the desired site and contrast medium inserted. Serial radiographs are obtained. Due to the risk inherent in entering blood vessels, especially arteries, other procedures precede angiography in the diagnostic process. This procedure is contraindicated during pregnancy.

Nursing Interventions: Client education includes an explanation of the procedure and emphasis on remaining still during the procedure. Children may require sedation or restraint. Clients are told that injection of contrast medium may provoke an unpleasant feeling. Clients are told in advance of the routine postprocedure monitoring. A client history specific for pregnancy and prior allergic response to contrast medium is obtained. Adequacy of clotting status is determined. Anticoagulant therapy may be temporarily interrupted. The client is NPO past midnight prior to the exam to reduce the risk of reaction to contrast medium. The client wears a hospital gown, and removes all jewelry and prostheses.

Description of the Procedure: This procedure is performed with inpatients and outpatients when sufficient postprocedure monitoring is available. The client goes to an x-ray room. The entry site is prepared. Local anesthesia is administered and the entry site draped. The client is instructed not to move until visualization is complete. A catheter is inserted and threaded via fluoroscopy to the desired site. Contrast medium is inserted through the catheter and serial timed radiographs obtained. Many clients report discomfort, associated with catheter manipulation or contrast insertion, during this procedure. The catheter is withdrawn. Sutures or dressings may be applied to the entry site. Renal angiography takes approximately 1–2 hours. Preliminary results may be available immediately, but final interpretation follows detailed viewing of the films.

Evaluating Client Response: Following the procedure, the client is supine with the entry site immobilized. Pressure, by sandbag or dressing, may be applied. The insertion site is checked for signs of bleeding. Arterial pulses, skin color and temperature distal to the insertion site are closely monitored. Vital signs are taken every 15 minutes for the first 4 hours, every 30 minutes for the next 2 hours, and every 4 hours prn. Voiding is monitored. Food and medications are resumed. Fluid intake is encouraged to promote excretion of the contrast medium. Analgesics are administered as needed. Outpatients should not drive themselves home. Client and family support in dealing with the results is provided.

DIRECT VISUALIZATION

- **Urethroscopy**
- **Percutaneous Nephroscopy**

The direct visualization of the bladder, urethra, and kidneys by insertion of a cystoscope is termed enduroscopy. Renal visualization may also be performed percutaneously. A specific consent form may be required for these procedures.

Nursing Diagnoses for clients undergoing direct visualization include:

- Alteration in comfort related to procedure
- Anxiety related to procedure
- Knowledge deficit related to diagnostic process
- Potential for injury related to procedure
- Potential for infection related to procedure

Urethroscopy (Cystoscopy, Nephroscopy)

Subjective Data: Client complains of pain, frequency, or difficulty voiding.

Objective Data: Altered physical findings, repeated urinary problems and abnormal laboratory analyses of blood and/or urine.

Assessment: Urethroscopy permits direct examination of the urethra for strictures or bleeding sites. Cystoscopy, using either a rigid or a flexible cystoscope, is used to examine clients with suspected bleeding, calculi, fistula, or tumor. In addition, cystoscopy is used to collect urine directly from a kidney, measure bladder capacity, test for vesicoureteral reflex, or biopsy the bladder or urethra. Using a flexible, fiberoptic cystoscope, nephroscopy allows direct visualization of the renal pelvis, calyces, fundus, and collecting system. Nephroscopy is used for diagnostic assessment of calculi or hematuria and for renal brush biopsy as well as for surgical removal of calculi or tumor resection. Diagnostically, these procedures are most commonly performed with local anesthesia, although most surgical visualizations are done with general anesthesia.

Nursing Interventions: Client education includes an explanation of the procedure and instructions regarding positioning, remaining still, and postprocedure fluid intake, and urine color changes. The client is prepared to expect some postprocedure discomfort. Urethroscopies performed with younger children commonly require general anesthesia. The ability of the older child to cooperate during the procedure forms the basis for the general-versus-local-anesthesia decision. Client preparation varies widely with the institution and the individual purpose of the procedure. Some clients are NPO and receive sedatives prior to this procedure. Some clients receive general anesthesia and all safety precautions and associated nursing responsibilities are implemented. Other clients receive oral or IV sedation during the procedure. Local anesthetic may be applied at the time of cystoscope insertion. Some clients receive enemas to clear the bowel. If present during cystoscopy, the nurse provides client reassurance and technical assistance.

Description of the Procedure: These procedures are performed with inpatients and outpatients. The client assumes the lithotomy position. With sterile technique, the cystoscope is inserted into the urethra and advanced into the bladder. In order to avoid trauma to the urinary tract, it is essential the client remain still during the procedure. The client may experience some pressure or pain sensations as the scope is advanced and rotated. Sterile irrigating solution may be inserted to distend the bladder for complete visualization. When the procedure is completed, any fluid inserted is removed and the cystoscope is withdrawn. Length of time for the procedure depends on what is done during cystoscopy and ranges from 10 minutes to 2 hours. The results of visualization are available immediately; results of biopsies or other tests requiring laboratory analysis take longer to obtain.

Evaluating Client Response: Clients who have received general anesthesia receive appropriate postsurgical nursing care. For all clients, vital signs are monitored. Following cystoscopy, some blood-tinged urine is expected. Copious bleeding or clots are considered adverse reactions and the physician is notified. Back pain, bladder spasms, and feelings of burning and fullness are expected. Moist heat, warm baths, or analgesia are administered as appropriate. The client is monitored for urinary retention. Food and medications are resumed. Fluid intake is encouraged to dilute the urine and reduce irritation of the urinary tract. If dyes were administered as part of the procedure, the urine will be discolored. Some clients experience postprocedure chilling with a slight rise in temperature. If these symptoms do not subside with rest, warmth, and fluids, the physician is notified. Postprocedure client and family support is provided.

■ Percutaneous Nephroscopy

Subjective Data: See preceding section for urethroscopy.

Objective Data: See preceding section for urethroscopy.

Assessment: The renal pelvis, calyces, fundus, and collecting system may be examined by percutaneous insertion of a fiberoptic nephroscope.

Nursing Intervention: See following section for renal biopsy.

Description of the Procedure: Ultrasonography, fluoroscopy, or CT is used as guide during needle insertion. Initially, a needle is placed into the renal collecting system and a flexible guide wire advanced through this needle. A series of dilators is passed to widen the nephrocutaneous tract. Once the tract is enlarged, a rigid or flexible fiberoptic endoscope is advanced through the tract in order to visualize the intrarenal collecting system. This procedure is used to locate calculi and determine the site of bleeding. This procedure can also be used to remove stones 1.5 cm or smaller.

Evaluating Client Response: See following section for renal biopsy.

■ PERCUTANEOUS RENAL BIOPSY

Bladder and retrograde brush renal biopsy are performed during cystoscopy and are discussed in the previous section. Renal biopsy is a major, invasive procedure. A specific consent form is required.

Nursing Diagnoses for clients undergoing renal biopsy include:

- Alteration in comfort related to procedure
- Anxiety related to procedure
- Knowledge deficit related to diagnostic process
- Potential for injury: bleeding related to procedure

Subjective Data: Client complains of pain, tenderness, malaise, and weakness.

Objective Data: Abnormal physical findings indicative of electrolyte imbalance such as edema, nausea, vomiting, or fatigue, and abnormal laboratory data.

Assessment: Renal biopsies are performed by needle aspiration, either percutaneously or via a small flank incision. Due to the vascularity of the kidneys, potential postprocedure bleeding is a major concern. Therefore, biopsies are performed on clients whose clotting profile, blood type, and cross-match have been determined. Percutaneous renal biopsies are not performed on clients with only one functioning kidney.

Nursing Interventions: Client education includes an explanation of the procedure, emphasizing the need to remain still and hold one's breath. Children may require additional assistance during this procedure. The client is prepared for postprocedure monitoring and activity restrictions. Determination of current clotting profile, and blood typing and cross-matching if ordered, is made. Clients are NPO 6–8 hours prior to renal biopsy. Sedation is administered and an IV line is established before the biopsy. If present during the procedure, the nurse helps the client remain still, provides emotional support, and technical assistance as needed.

Description of the Procedure: Renal biopsies are done with inpatients and outpatients when sufficient postprocedure monitoring is available. Baseline vital signs and a urine sample are obtained. Fluoroscopy or ultrasound may be used to position the needle. The client is placed in a prone position, with a sandbag under the abdomen. The entry site is located and prepared and local anesthetic is administered. The client is told to take a deep breath and hold the inspiration to immobilize the kidney. Using sterile technique, the aspiration needle is inserted into the outer quadrant of the kidney and aspirated and then withdrawn. Following the procedure, pressure is applied to the insertion site and the client is kept supine. The procedure is completed in less than 10 minutes. The results are available following laboratory analysis.

Evaluating Client Response: Vital signs are monitored every 10–15 minutes for the first hour, and 30 minutes for 1 hour, every 1 hour for 2 hours, every 2 hours for 2 hours and every 4 hours overnight. The client is assessed for bleeding at the entry site, pain, and urinary status. The client lies flat on his or her back for 4 hours and is then on bed rest for 8–12 hours. Changes in blood pressure, anorexia, abdominal discomfort, backache, shoulder pain, or dysuria may be signs of bleeding in the kidney and are reported to the physician. All urine is compared to the preprocedure sample and is examined for blood. Food and medications are resumed. Fluid intake is encouraged to avoid clot formation and retention. Clients are advised to avoid strenuous activity for several days. Outpatients should not drive themselves home. Client and family support in dealing with the results is provided as needed.

7

Clients with Impaired Mobility

Clients with impaired mobility may have dysfunction in the musculoskeletal system or the central or peripheral nervous systems. Impaired mobility may also be secondary to pathophysiology elsewhere in the body. Impaired mobility may result from different sources including external or internal physical or chemical insult, infection, degenerative disease, neoplasm, or biochemical defect. Any associated impairment in ability to perform activities of daily living results in major changes in the life style of client and family. The process of determining the cause of neuroskeletalmuscular defects may be arduous and taxing for the client. Nursing diagnoses address psychosocial needs in addition to pathophysiologic concerns.

For clients with impaired mobility, physical examination provides diagnostic data and information about how pathophysiology is affecting the client's life style. The joints, spine, muscles, peripheral nerves, central nervous system, client's mental status, and life style are assessed, as are other interrelated glands and tissues. Physical assessment includes a detailed recording of the client's subjective complaints and history of the present illness. In addition, information about the client's personal and family history are obtained. Physical examination of the client with impaired mobility may be lengthy and repeated frequently, even daily, to assess changes brought about by disease or treatment. Client cooperation and comfort during the examination contribute greatly it its accuracy.

LABORATORY TESTS

Clients can develop impaired mobility from a wide variety of pathophysiologic sources. Drug toxicology testing is included in this section, as drug-related response must be considered when clients present with neurologic changes. Client cooperation enhances the efficient use of time, resources, and money during the diagnostic process.

Nursing Diagnoses for clients undergoing laboratory tests include:

- Anxiety related to procedure
- Knowledge deficit related to diagnostic process

LABORATORY TESTS

Test	Purpose	Normal Values	Nursing Actions
Antinuclear antibodies (ANA) Serum	Assess for lupus erythematosus, systemic sclerosis, rheumatoid or juvenile arthritis, diabetic status	Negative Titer: <1:10	
Cholinesterase RBC Serum	Assess effect of muscle relaxants, monitor for poisoning	8–18 μml	
HLA-B27 HLA-TMO Serum	Assess for juvenile arthritis	Negative	
Hydroxyproline Urine	Assess bone reabsorption, Paget's disease, bone tumors	Total: 22–27 μg/24 hr Free: <2 mg/24 hr	Collection container must contain preservative and be refrigerated
Phenylketonuria test (PKU) Blood	Determine presence of phenylalanine,	<4 mg/100 ml within 4 days of birth	

(Continued)

LABORATORY TESTS (cont.)

Test	Purpose	Normal Values	Nursing Actions
PKU (*cont.*) Urine	PKU disease. Routine screening test for newborns	Negative several wk after birth	
Rheumatoid factor (RA factor, rheumaton, latex fixation) Serum	Assess for lupus erythematosus	Negative or <1:20	
Vitamin D and metabolites Serum	Assess nutritional status, calcium homostasis	Winter: 14–42 ng/ml Summer: 15–80 ng/ml 25-(OH)D3: 15–155 ng/ml 1,25-(OH)D3: 20–76 pg/ml	

Please note, these values are guidelines. Check with the laboratory performing the test for absolute values.

DRUG LEVELS

Drug	Effective Concentrations	Nursing Actions
Alcohol ethanol	Legal toxicity varies, may begin at 0.05–0.15 g/100 ml	
Acetaminophen	Therapeutic: 10–20 μg/ml Toxic: >300 μg/ml	
Barbiturate	Therapeutic: Adult and Child: Phenobarbital: 1.5–4.0 mg/100 ml Others: 0.05–0.3 mg/100 ml Toxic: Adult and Child: Short-acting: 3 mg/100 ml Moderate-acting: 6 mg/100 ml Long-acting: 9 mg/100 ml	
Cadmium	Normal:	
Serum	Negative	
Urine	<15 μg/24 hr	
Carbamazepine	Therapeutic: 3–9 μg/ml	
Carbon monoxide	0–2% saturation. Symptoms appear with levels over 20%	
Chlordiazepoxide	Therapeutic: 1–3 μg/ml	
Chlorpromazine	Therapeutic:	

DRUG LEVELS (cont.)

Drug	Effective Concentrations	Nursing Actions
Chlorpromazine (*cont.*)	Adult: 30–50 ng/ml Children: 40–80 ng/ml	
Clonazepam	Therapeutic: 5–70 ng/ml	
Desipramine	Therapeutic: 40–60 ng/ml Toxic: >1 μg/ml	
Diazepam	Therapeutic: 300–400 ng/ml	
Diphenhydramine	Therapeutic: >25 ng/ml Toxic: >100 μg/ml	
Doxepin	Therapeutic: 30–150 ng/ml	
Ethosuximide	Therapeutic: 40–100 μg/ml	
Haloperidol	Therapeutic: 1 ng/ml Toxic: >15 ng/ml	
Imipramine	Therapeutic: 100–300 ng/ml Toxic: >1 μg/ml	
Indomethacin	Therapeutic: 0.3–3 μg/ml Toxic: >5 μg/ml	
Lead	Normal: negative	
Serum	Toxic: >0.08 mg/100 ml	
Urine	>0.08 mg/24 hr	Collection container must contain preservative or be kept on ice
Lithium	Therapeutic: 0.6–1.2 mEq/L Toxic: >2.0 mEq/L	
Meperidine	Therapeutic: 0.4–0.7 μg/ml	
Methanol	May be fatal when as low as 10 mg/100 ml	
Methsuximide	Therapeutic: 10–100 μg/ml	
Naproxen	Therapeutic: >50 μg/ml	
Nitrazepam	Toxic: >200 ng/ml	
Nortriptyline	Therapeutic: 50–140 ng/ml	
Phensuximide	Therapeutic: 40–80 μg/ml	
Phenylbutazone	Therapeutic: 50–150 μg/ml	
Phenytoin	Therapeutic: 10–20 μg/100 ml	
Primidone	Therapeutic: 4–12 μg/ml	
Protriptyline	Therapeutic: 100–200 ng/100 ml	
Pyridostigmine	Therapeutic: 50–100 ng/ml	
Salicylate	Therapeutic: 150–300 μg/ml	Draw specimen 2 hr after dose
Trimethadione	Therapeutic: 20–40 μg/ml	
Valproic acid	Therapeutic: 50–100 μg/ml	

Please note, these values are guidelines. Check with the laboratory performing the test for absolute values.

ULTRASONOGRAPHY

Echoencephalography is ultrasound of the brain. No specific consent form is required.

Nursing Diagnoses for clients undergoing these procedures include:

- Anxiety related to procedure
- Knowledge deficit related to the diagnostic process

Subjective Data: Client complains of headaches, dizziness, syncope, or changes in vision.

Objective Data: Altered mental status exam, lethargy, irritability, restlessness, vision or pupillary changes, and vomiting.

Assessment: Echoencephalography provides for a rapid determination of the position of midline structures and thus is used to evaluate the presence of subdural hematoma, intracerebral hemorrhage, massive cerebral infarct or neoplasm. The width of the lateral ventricles can be evaluated as can shifts of the ventricles associated with expanding lesions. Echoencephalography is particularly useful in infants and neonates due to the presence of relatively more fluid in the subarachnoid space and the higher water content of the brain. In infants, the brain is measured along with assessment for hydrocephalus, intracranial hemorrhage, congenital anomalies, or tumors. A real-time scanner can be used at the bedside, whereas a static water bath scanner allows the infant to be positioned but not touched by the transducer. Doppler ultrasonography is a frequently used tool for assessing the carotid bifurcation and patency of the carotid arteries. Doppler ultrasound is used as a diagnostic procedure and to follow the client's disease course and/or response to therapy. Ultrasonography has limited use in examining other body parts that may be involved in clients with impaired mobility.

Nursing Interventions: Client education includes an explanation of the procedure. Specific instructions are provided regarding remaining still and feeling some pressure during the procedure. To relax infants, ultrasound is performed after the baby has eaten and is comfortable. If a water bath is used, the water is set at body temperature to prevent hypothermia.

Description of the Procedure: This procedure is performed with inpatients and outpatients. Echoencephalography requires a quiet, nonstimulating environment in order to discourage movement. When a real-time scanner is used, conductive oil or gel is applied to the scanning site for optimal contact between transducer and skin. The transducer is moved across the skull. Static water bath scanners, however, require only correct positioning of the infant. For Doppler ultrasound, the client is recumbent and relaxed. Ultrasound examinations take less than 30 minutes to complete. The results are available following interpretation.

Evaluating Client Response: If needed, assistance is provided to help the client remove any oil or gel. Client and family support is provided.

OCULAR PLETHYSMOGRAPHY (OPG, OCULAR PNEUMOPLETHYSMOGRAPHY, OPG-GEE)

Plethysmography records eye volume changes as a means of evaluating blood flow in the carotid arteries. A specific consent form may be required.

Nursing Diagnoses for clients undergoing OPG include:

- Alteration in comfort related to procedure
- Anxiety related to procedure
- Knowledge deficit related to diagnostic process

Subjective Data: Client complains of dizziness, syncope, or blurred vision.

Objective Data: Altered physical findings including carotid bruits, altered neurologic exam, and changes in sensory and motor function.

Assessment: OPG is used to diagnose, locate, screen, and follow occlusive disease and response to therapy in the left and right internal and external carotid arteries. A pressure difference of more than 5 between eyes is considered clinically significant. The results of this test are frequently combined with the results from ultrasonography in determining client treatment. Clients with negative results from both tests do not need angiography. OPG is contraindicated within 6 months of most forms of eye surgery, in clients with glaucoma, or with a history of surgical lens implantation or retinal detachment.

Nursing Interventions: Client education includes an explanation of the procedure. Clients are prepared for and reassured about eye dryness and redness. A client history specific for prior eye disorders and treatment is obtained. Eye glasses and contact lenses are removed.

Description of the Procedure: OPG is performed with inpatients and outpatients. The client is supine and made comfortable. Local anesthetic may be placed on the sclerae. Suction cups are placed on the outer portion of the sclerae and eye volumes are recorded. OPG may also include applying pressure to the eyes and recording the responses. Recording existing pressure takes less than 1 minute, but recording responses to pressure will take longer. The results are available immediately.

Evaluating Client Response: Clients frequently report feeling dryness in the eyes for the rest of the day and may have redness at the site of eye cup application for up to 3 days. Neither of these is considered clinically significant. Methylcellulose drops may be used to ease dryness. Client and family are reassured about these sequellae.

MEASUREMENT OF ELECTRICAL ACTIVITY

- **Electromyography**
- **Electroencephalography**

These procedures provide graphic recordings of electrical activity within skeletal muscles and the brain respectively. These tests detect electrical abnormalities that may be indicative of pathophysiologic states. A specific consent form may be required.

Nursing Diagnoses include:

- Anxiety related to procedure
- Alteration in comfort related to procedure
- Knowledge deficit related to diagnostic process

Electromyography (EMG, Nerve Conduction Study)

Subjective Data: Client complains of weakness and pain.

Objective Data: Changes in muscle function as evidenced by muscle weakness, difficulty with voluntary movement, etc.

Assessment: EMG provides data about electrical activity within the motor unit of skeletal muscles. Needle electrodes are inserted into the muscle and the electrical activity is displayed on an oscilloscope, heard via a loudspeaker and/or recorded. Each motor unit is measured to identify or rule out a characteristic altered pattern of activity. EMG is used to determine neuromuscular disorders and myopathies. Medication effectiveness, time and manner of reinnervation of muscles, and aberrant conduction velocities can also be determined.

Nursing Interventions: Client education includes an explanation of the procedure and the importance of client cooperation. The client is prepared for needle insertion, contracting and relaxing muscles upon request, and seeing and hearing the results. Postprocedure muscle soreness and the availability of analgesia are discussed. Clients may be asked to avoid caffeine and cigarettes for 2–4 hours prior to this test. Premedication is avoided to ensure that the client can comply with directions during this somewhat uncomfortable procedure.

Description of the Procedure: EMG is performed on inpatients and outpatients. The client goes to the examining room. Thin needle electrodes are inserted into the muscle to be tested. Electrical activity is recorded at the time of needle insertion, immediately afterward, with the muscle at rest, and with minimal and maximal muscle contraction, as performed by the client upon request. Nerve conduction studies are performed by stimulating a peripheral nerve, usng a surface electrode, and recording the response of the muscle. The needles are then removed. The time needed for an EMG depends upon how many muscles are being studied. The results are available following interpretation.

Evaluating Client Response: Postprocedure muscle soreness is expected. Analgesics are administered as needed. Client and family support in dealing with the procedure and the results is provided.

■ Electroencephalography (EEG, Evoked Potential Studies, Visual Evoked Potential, VEP, Auditory Brain Stem Response, ABR)

Subjective Data: Client complains of headaches, dizziness, syncope, or aura.

Objective Data: The presence of seizures, altered levels of consciousness, loss of muscle tone, abnormal respiratory pattern.

Assessment: EEGs are used to assess intracranial pathophysiology, to determine the presence of and type of epilepsy, and to assess organic brain syndrome. EEGs are also used to determine brain death. An EEG demonstrates the frequency, amplitude, and type of brain waves present. In a normal EEG, there is symmetry of alpha, beta, and delta waves. VEP studies are used in clients who cannot or will not cooperate with subjective testing and primarily reflect central visual function, especially visual acuity. ABR studies reflect 8th cranial nerve function.

Nursing Interventions: Client education includes an explanation of the procedure, the need to lie still, and the availability of rest periods. The client is prepared to be alone in a darkened room with the technician on the other side of a window but in voice and sight contact with the client at all times. Children under 18 months of age may need to be sedated. Stimulants and depressants, including alcohol, coffee, tea, and cola drinks are not allowed the day of the EEG. Ideally, anticonvulsants are withheld for 48 hours prior to this procedure. Nevertheless, client status frequently makes this unfeasible. Unless a sleep recording is desired, sedation is withheld for 6–8 hours prior to the procedure.

Description of the Procedure: The procedure is performed on inpatients and outpatients. Bedside EEGs are most commonly used to determine brain death. Otherwise, the client goes to a room specially shielded to eliminate outside electrical interference and other disruptions. During the

EEG, the client is alone in the room but can see the technician through a window. Sixteen to thirty-two electrodes are applied with electrode paste over corresponding sides of the head. One electrode may be placed on each earlobe for grounding. The client must lie perfectly still. This procedure is tiring for the client and breaks in recording are taken every 5 minutes to allow the client to move and stretch as desired. EEGs may include asking the client to hyperventilate at a rate of 30–40 breaths per minute for 3 minutes. The resulting alkalosis will accentuate any abnormal brain activity. Evoked potential studies may be part of an EEG.

For VEP studies, electrodes are placed over the occipital cortex. A visual stimulus, such as flashing strobe light, is presented to the client. For ABR, an auditory stimulus, such as a clicking sound, is used. The changes in waves that occur are used to assess cranial nerve and/or brain functioning. EEGs take approximately 1 hour to complete. Sleep EEGs take approximately 3 hours to complete. The results are available following interpretation.

Evaluating Client Response: Following the procedure, the client receives assistance as needed in getting all of the electrode paste out of the hair. Client and family support in dealing with the results is provided.

THERMOGRAPHY

Thermography uses a heat-sensitive camera to measure heat radiating from the surface of the skin. Interpretation of the results provides data regarding circulation to and tissue distribution within the photographed area. A specific consent form is not required.

Nursing Diagnoses for clients undergoing thermography include:

- Anxiety related to procedure
- Knowledge deficit related to diagnostic process

Subjective Data: Client complains of pain and difficulty with activities of daily living.

Objective Data: Altered joint appearance and mobility.

Assessment: Thermography is used to assess clients with suspected joint disease, especially rheumatoid arthritis, and to assess client response to drug therapy. There is some use of thermographic techniques to assess facial and scalp pain.

Nursing Interventions: Client education includes specific instructions for remaining still during the procedure. Discussion may emphasize the short time period required for photography, particularly if the client is experiencing joint discomfort.

Description of the Procedure: This procedure is performed with inpatients and outpatients. The client is positioned so that the desired joint is partially flexed and the maximum joint surface can be photographed. This may cause some client discomfort. Several photographs of each joint may be obtained from different angles. Thermography takes less than 15 minutes to complete. The results are available following interpretation.

Evaluating Client Response: Analgesia is administered as needed. Client and family support is provided.

MAGNETIC RESONANCE IMAGING (NUCLEAR MAGNETIC IMAGING, MR, NMR)

Magnetic resonance imaging is a noninvasive method of assessing tissue composition. This technique has shown its greatest potential for clients with impaired mobility. A specific consent form may be required.

Nursing Diagnoses for the client undergoing MR include:

- Anxiety related to procedure
- Knowledge deficit related to diagnostic process

Subjective Data: Client complains of sensory or motor difficulty, dizziness, syncope, and/or pain.

Objective Data: Changes in mental status, neurologic or sensory examinations, and abnormal results from other diagnostic testing.

Assessment: For clients with impaired mobility, MR has two distinct uses, imaging and describing specific chemical composition. Thus, in addition to defining anatomy, MR can define changes in tissue metabolism. MR provides excellent contrast in imaging the soft tissues in extremities and is being used to distinguish benign and malignant lesions. The medullary cavity of bones visualizes well, due to the high fat content of marrow. MR is preferable to CT for clients who require imaging of the posterior fossa or when a high level of contrast between gray and white matter is desired. MR is used to assess clients with suspected intracranial disease, hemorrhage, mass, or lesion, cerebral infarct hydrocephalus, hematoma, aneurysm, or lesions caused by multiple sclerosis and other demyelinating diseases. Interpretation of pediatric MR of the brain is being refined. MR can also identify abnormalities of the craniovertebral junction. It is used to assess clients with suspected syringohydromyelia, intramedullary spinal cord tumors, neurofibroma, lipoma, spinal dysxaphism, trauma, marrow replacement disease, or intervertebral disc disease with or without herniation. The pituitary gland also visualizes well. MR is contraindicated in clients with aneurysm clips anywhere in the body or with pacemakers because of the effects of the magnetic field.

Nursing Interventions: Client education includes the need to remain still during imaging. The ability of children to cooperate is determined. Sedation and restraints are usually required for infants and very young children. Clients are prepared for the imposing size of the MR scanner and the noninvasive nature of the procedure is emphasized. A client history specific for the presence of aneurysm clips or a pacemaker is obtained. The client changes into a hospital gown and removes all jewelry and prostheses.

Description of the Procedure: This procedure is performed with inpatients and outpatients. The client goes to the MR room. The client is supine within the body scanner during the scanning procedure. Completion time depends upon image quality and takes approximately 45 minutes. Results are available after interpretation.

Evaluating Client Response: Postprocedure client and family support is provided.

SCINTIGRAPHY

- **Synovial Scintigraphy**
- **Bone Scan**
- **Photon Absorptiometry**
- **Brain Scan**
- **Cerebral Blood Flow Study**
- **Radioisotope Angiogram**
- **Cisternal Scan**

For clients with impaired mobility, scintigraphic studies provide data about the brain, bones, and joints. Tumors, abscesses and hematomas can be detected. The use of various types of brain scintigraphy along with computed tomography have resulted in the almost total decline of pneumoencephalography. A specific consent form may be required for these procedures.

Nursing Diagnoses for clients undergoing scintigraphy include:

- Alteration in comfort related to procedure
- Anxiety related to procedure
- Knowledge deficit related to diagnostic procedure

■ Synovial Scintigraphy

Subjective Data: Client complains of pain, recent trauma, or changes in mobility.

Objective Data: Swelling, changes in configuration, and redness.

Assessment: This study is used to detect polyarthritis, osteoarthritis, ankylosing spondylitis, and other causes of arthritis. Tc-99m-labeled radionuclides are most commonly used. Scintigraphy is contraindicated during pregnancy and lactation.

Nursing Interventions: Client education includes an explanation of the procedure, the need for total rest of the affected joint for 1 hour prior to injection, and positioning. Children may require additional assistance during this procedure. A client history specific for pregnancy and previous reaction to contrast media is obtained. Potential cross-interference is reduced by allowing 24–48 hours to separate different nuclear medicine studies.

Description of the Procedure: This procedure is performed with inpatients and outpatients. The client may be asked to rest the affected joint totally for 1 hour prior to the test. The client receives an IV injection of the radiopharmaceutical and joint imaging starts immediately. This procedure is completed in less than 45 minutes. The results are available following interpretation.

Evaluating Client Response: Postprocedure support for client and family in dealing with the results is provided.

■ Bone Scan (Skeletal Survey)

Subjective Data: Client complains of pain or changes in mobility.

Objective Data: Altered neuromuscular exam, known neoplastic disease, fever, or abnormal results from laboratory tests and/or x-rays.

Assessment: Bone scans are used to detect metastasis, infectious states such as osteomyelitis and tuberculosis, metabolic diseases such as Paget's disease, parathyroid disorders, and pathologic and traumatic fractures. Bone scans are also used to stage, determine therapy, and response to therapy in clients with carcinoma. Various radionuclides are in use, most commonly Tc-99m-labeled compounds. Scintigraphy is contraindicated during pregnancy and lactation.

Nursing Interventions: Client education includes an explanation of the procedure and the possibility of repeated imaging. Children may require additional assistance during this procedure. A client history specific for pregnancy and previous reaction to contrast media is obtained. Potential cross-interference is reduced by allowing 24–48 hours to separate different nuclear medicine studies. Clients are well-hydrated prior to this procedure. All jewelry and prostheses are removed and the client voids before going to the nuclear medicine department.

Description of the Procedure: This procedure is performed with inpatients and outpatients. The client receives an IV injection of radiopharmaceutical approximately 2–3 hours before imaging. The client's position depends on which body part is being scanned. Imaging may be repeated at various intervals. Skeletal imaging may be repeated up to 24 hours later. This procedure requires 45–60 minutes for each imaging session. The results are available following interpretation.

Evaluating Client Response: The client is encouraged to drink fluids to aid in urinary excretion of the radionuclide. Postprocedure support for client and family in dealing with the results is provided.

■ Photon Absorptiometry (Norland–Cameron Single Photon Absorptiometry, Dual Photon Absorptiometry, Bone Density Test)

Subjective Data: Client complains of pain or changes in mobility.

Objective Data: Changes in posture and/or evidence of fracture on x-ray.

Assessment: Photon absorption studies are used to assess bone mass in clients with suspected osteoporosis. Norland-Cameron absorptiometry measures the mineral content of long bones. Dual photon absorptiometry permits differentiation of fat and soft, i.e., marrow tissue components of bone and is considered to be more accurate. It can be used for quantitative imaging of the axial skeleton. Results of these studies are based on interpretation of the passage of photons through the bone.

Nursing Interventions: Preprocedure nursing responsibilities include an explanation of the procedure.

Description of the Procedure: This procedure is performed with inpatients and outpatients. Clients go to a specific room for these studies. For Norland-Cameron absorptiometry, the forearm (or other bone) is encased in a tissue equivalent solution. The arm is then positioned with the radioactive iodine photon source below and the collimated scintillation camera above. The photon beam is measured as it passes through the arm. Dual photon absorptiometry uses a similar technique except that the radioisotope emits photons at two different energy levels in order to differentiate bone and marrow. These procedures are completed in less than 20 minutes. The results are available following interpretation.

Evaluating Client Response: Following the procedure, client and family support is provided.

■ Brain Scan

Subjective Data: Client complains of changes in mental status or mobility.

Objective Data: Altered neurologic or mental status exam, abnormal vision or gait, known neoplastic disease, abnormal results from other diagnostic tests.

Assessment: Brain scans are used when CT cannot be done or is normal or equivocal. Brain scans are used to delineate subdural hematoma, arteriovenous malformation, cerebral thrombosis, brain abscess, vascular neoplasm, malignant glioma, and many other types of metastatic tumors. After infarction, areas of enhancement or abnormal uptake are evidenced in 2–7 days, become increasingly concentrated for 2–3 weeks and then subside. In several months, the brain scan returns to normal. Scintigraphy is contraindicated during pregnancy and lactation.

Nursing Interventions: Client education includes an explanation of the procedure and the timing involved. The client is prepared to receive oral and IV radiopharmaceuticals. Children may require additional assistance during this procedure. A client history specific for pregnancy and previous reaction to contrast media is obtained. Potential cross-interference is reduced by allowing 24–48 hours to separate different nuclear medicine studies.

Description of the Procedure: This procedure is performed with inpatients and outpatients. The client receives a blocking agent, most commonly potassium perchlorate 600 mg, to block uptake of the radioisotope by the thyroid, choroid plexus, salivary glands, and oropharyngeal mucosa. The client receives an IV injection of the radiopharmaceutical 15–30 minutes later. Imaging with a contact scanner takes place immediately after injection and again in 2 hours. This procedure requires 30–45 minutes for each imaging and is completed in approximately 3 hours. The results are available following interpretation.

Evaluating Client Response: Following the procedure, the client is encouraged to drink fluids to aid in excretion of the radioisotope. Postprocedure support for client and family in dealing with the results is provided.

■ Cerebral Blood Flow Study (Regional Cerebral Blood Flow Study)

Subjective Data: Client complains of changes in mental status.

Objective Data: Altered neurologic or mental status exam, altered vision or gait, previous transient ischemic attack (TIA).

Assessment: This test measures blood flow through the cerebral vasculature and thus provides an estimate of cerebral perfusion. Clients with suspected TIA may undergo repetitive studies to predict the danger of infarction and along with other tests determine if intracranial bypass surgery might be beneficial. This procedure is also used to assess response to therapy of clients who are hypertensive and to evaluate the effects of surgery. This is a noninvasive study in which the client inhales Xe-131 and electrodes are used to detect its presence in the cerebral circulation. Occasionally, this test is performed with intracarotid artery injection of the radiopharmaceutical. The normal Xe-131 diffusion rate is 56–91 ml/min/100 g. The normal isotope clearance rate is 50/ml/min/g. Scintigraphy is contraindicated during pregnancy and lactation.

Nursing Interventions: Client education includes an explanation of the procedure. The use of the mask or mouthpiece and nose clips or intracarotid artery injection is explained as appropriate. All hair clips, etc., are removed. Central nervous system stimulants and depressants may be withheld for 24 hours prior to the procedure. A client history specific for pregnancy is obtained. Potential cross-interference is reduced by allowing 24–48 hours to separate different nuclear medicine studies.

Description of the Procedure: This procedure is performed with inpatients and outpatients. Intracarotid-injection studies are usually performed with inpatients. The client goes to the Nuclear Medicine Department where 16–32 detectors are placed on the client's scalp. For an inhalation study, the client sits and uses either a mask or a mouthpiece and nose clips. The client inhales Xe-131 deeply through the mouth for 1 minute and then inhales room air for 10 minutes. For injection studies, the client is supine and one or both carotid arteries are used. Pressure dressings are applied immediately to the puncture sites. For each study, the flow rate and clearance rates are recorded following administration of the radioisotope. This procedure is completed in approximately 30 minutes. The results are available following interpretation.

Evaluating Client Response: Following a noninvasive cerebral blood flow study, the client requires no specific monitoring. Following intracarotid injection, however, the client is maintained on bed rest with the head elevated for 4–12 hours. The injection sites are monitored for bleeding; neurologic and vital signs are obtained every 15 minutes the first hour, every 30 minutes the second hour, and every hour thereafter until stable. An ice collar is applied. Fluids are provided as client status permits. Client and family support is provided.

■ Radioisotope Angiogram

Subjective Data: Client complains of changes in mental status.

Objective Data: Altered neurologic or mental status exam, changes in vision or gait, abnormal findings from other diagnostic testing.

Assessment: This study demonstrates blood flow through the brain. The client receives a bolus of Te-99m intravenously. The resulting isotope course is visualized by a gamma camera. Normally, there is simultaneous transit through the two carotid arteries and anterior and middle cerebral arteries. Scintigraphy is contraindicated during pregnancy and lactation.

Nursing Interventions: Client education includes an explanation of the procedure. Children may require additional assistance during this procedure. A client history specific for pregnancy and previous reaction to contrast media is obtained. Potential cross-interference is reduced by allowing 24–48 hours to separate different nuclear medicine studies.

Description of the Procedure: This procedure is performed with inpatients and outpatients. In the Nuclear Medicine Department, the client assumes a supine position. The radiopharmaceutical is injected intravenously and imaging begins immediately. This procedure is completed in approximately 30 minutes. The results are available following interpretation.

Evaluating Client Response: Following the procedure, the client is encouraged to drink fluids to aid in excretion of the radioisotope. Postprocedure support for client and family in dealing with the results is provided.

■ Cisternal Scan

Subjective Data: Client complains of changes in mental status.

Objective Data: Altered neurologic or mental status exam, changes in vision or gait, fever, abnormal findings from other diagnostic testing.

Assessment: Cisternal scans are performed to evaluate ventricular size, the patency of CSF pathways, and reabsorption. Cisternal scans can also detect the site of CSF leakage in clients with recurrent meningitis. Scintigraphy is contraindicated during pregnancy and lactation.

Nursing Interventions: Client education includes an explanation of the procedure and administration of the radiopharmaceutical. The possibility of repeated imaging is discussed. Children may require additional assistance during this procedure. A client history specific for pregnancy and previous reaction to contrast media is obtained. Potential crossinterference is reduced by allowing 24–48 hours to separate different nuclear medicine studies.

Description of the Procedure: This procedure is usually performed with inpatients. In the Nuclear Medicine Department, the client is positioned prone on the examining table. The lumbar entry site is located and prepared. The radiopharmaceutical is injected into the subarachnoid space and the needle withdrawn. Imaging begins immediately and may be repeated several times during a 24 to 72 hour period. The entry site is covered with a pressure bandage. The initial procedure is completed in approximately 30 minutes. The results are available following interpretation.

Evaluating Client Response: The client's neurologic status and vital signs are monitored every 15 minutes the first hour, every 30 minutes the next hour, and every hour thereafter until stable. Clients are maintained on bed rest for 4–12 hours. The entry site is monitored for signs of bleeding or leakage. The client is advised against overexertion for 24 hours. Client and family support in dealing with the results is provided.

RADIOLOGY

X-rays are a major diagnostic tool for clients with impaired mobility. A specific consent form may be required.

Nursing Diagnoses for clients undergoing x-rays include:

- Anxiety related to procedure
- Knowledge deficit related to diagnostic procedure

Subjective Data: Client complains of pain, recent trauma, or changes in mobility.

Objective Data: Evidence of trauma, decreased range of motion, or altered mental status exam.

Assessment: Radiographs of bone are used to determine bone density, texture, erosion, trauma, fracture, or new bone formation. Joint films are examined for evidence of osteoporosis, soft tissue swelling, calcification, joint space narrowing, subchondral cyst formation, or bony ankylosis. Clients with suspected arthritis undergo a radiographic series that includes both hands, knees, and two different views of the spine and pelvis. Spine and pelvic x-rays are contraindicated during pregnancy. For clients with suspected osteoporosis, diagnostic confirmation is obtained by calculating cortical thickness from a single plain radiograph of the hand. Clients with overt or suspected head trauma undergo a skull series to locate normally calcified structures such as the pineal body and choroid plexus, and to identify bony fractures, disruptions, distortions, or erosions. Specific views may be needed to assess the integrity of the facial bones.

Nursing Interventions: Nursing actions include an explanation of the procedure. Client transportation is appropriate to status. A client history specific as to pregnancy is obtained. Clients are encouraged to void before going to the radiology department. Clients who tend to chill easily may want additional blankets. The client wears a hospital gown. All jewelry and prostheses are removed.

Description of the Procedure: This procedure is performed on inpatients and outpatients. The client's position depends on the views to be obtained. Frequently, more than one radiograph is needed and the client may change position for each view. Clients receive instructions and assistance regarding the desired position and remaining still. In order to prevent any untoward effects on clients undergoing a skull series, the neck is never hyperextended, and manipulation is kept to a minimum. Each radiograph is completed in less than 5 minutes. The need for a series or for development of the x-rays before releasing the client may keep the client in the radiology department for 30–60 minutes. The results are available following interpretation.

Evaluating Client Response: Postprocedure support for client and family in dealing with the results is provided.

COMPUTED TOMOGRAPHY (CT, COMPUTERIZED AXIAL TOMOGRAPHY, CAT SCAN, EMI, COMPUTER ASSISTED MYELOGRAPHY, CAM, COMPUTED TOMOGRAPHY METRIZAMIDE MYELOGRAPHY, CTMM)

The technology of computed tomography is most widely applied to clients with problems of impaired mobility. CT scanning involves several views, but since scatter radiation is limited, the effects are not additive and each section receives only its own exposure. A specific consent form may be required.

Nursing Diagnoses for clients undergoing CT include:

- Anxiety related to procedure
- Knowledge deficit related to diagnostic process
- Potential for injury: allergic reaction related to procedure

Subjective Data: Client complains of pain, mood changes, and difficulty with activities of daily living.

Objective Data: Altered neuromuscular and mental status exams, changes in vision or gait.

Assessment: CT provides the basis for medical therapy for clients with complaints of back and neck pain. Contrast-enhanced CT is used to identify degenerative disorders of the spine including herniated or bulging disc, hypertrophic sparring, osteoarthritis of the facient joints, and lateral spinal stenosis. For clients with clinical evidence of osteoporosis, CT scans can be used to differentiate cortical and trabecular bone and to distinguish marrow from the mineral content of trabecular bone. CT is also used to identify soft tissue tumors and injury to ligaments and tendons, and to document injury in acutely traumatized children. CT may follow radiographs in an attempt to determine the presence of fracture in difficult-to-visualize areas. CT of the spine is contraindicated during pregnancy.

Cranial CT discriminates variations in tissue density and thus can differentiate hemorrhage, ischemia, and infarction and can exclude the presence of neoplasm or hematoma. CT is currently the primary diagnostic procedure for detecting intracranial mass, cerebral atrophy, hydrocephalus, and areas of cortical infarction. CT is used for infants to delineate developmental defects of the central nervous system. Contrast-enhanced CT scans are used to identify changes in tissue density and abnormal anatomic position of structures and blood vessels. Computer assisted myelography, CAM, involves intraspinal injection of the water soluble contrast medium, metrizamide. Cerebrospinal fluid spaces are evaluated and intradural lesions such as meningioma, neurofibroma, dermoid tumor, or ependynoma are identified.

Nursing Interventions: Client education prior to CT scanning includes an explanation of the procedure and the need to remain still during imaging. The ability of the child to cooperate by lying still and the need for sedation or restraint is determined. Some of the older CT scanners require up to 30 minutes and this may seem like a very long time to the client. The client is prepared for administration of the contrast medium. The imposing size of the CT scanner is explained and the noninvasive nature of the procedure is emphasized. If applicable, the technique of intraspinal injection is explained. A client history specific as to pregnancy is obtained. In addition, for contrast-enhanced scans, a history specific to allergy to iodine or previous reaction to contrast media is elicited. The specific procedure is explained to the client and family. Clients may be NPO 2–4 hours prior to contrast-enhanced scans, although clear liquids may be permitted. The client changes into a hospital gown, removes all jewelry and prostheses, voids, and goes to the CT room.

Description of the Procedure: CT is performed with inpatients and outpatients. The use and administration of contrast medium, either IV or intraspinal, depends on the type of scan being performed. Clients may experience a warm flushed feeling or a metallic taste in their mouths as the contrast medium is injected. The client is supine within the body scanner. For cranial scanning, the head is immobilized in a snug "cap." For spinal scanning, the client is positioned comfortably supine on the table with a bolster pillow between the knees. The client is asked to remain perfectly still during scanning. Cranial and spinal CT scans are completed in 15–30 minutes. Results are available after interpretation.

Evaluating Client Response: Food and medications are resumed. Fluid intake is encouraged to assist in eliminating the contrast medium and preventing dehydration. Postprocedure client and family support in dealing with the results is provided.

DIRECT VISUALIZATION

Arthroscopy is endoscopic direct visualization of a joint. A specific consent form may be required.

Nursing Diagnoses for clients undergoing arthroscopy include:

- Alteration in comfort related to procedure
- Anxiety related to diagnostic process
- Knowledge deficit related to procedure

Subjective Data: Client complains of pain or changes in mobility.

Objective Data: Altered physical exam, including swelling, discoloration, dislocation, or limited range of motion.

Assessment: Arthroscopy is most commonly performed on clients with disorders of the knee, such as traumatic injury or degenerative disease. Arthroscopy is frequently combined with arthrography and/or arthrocentesis to establish a definitive diagnosis. Arthroscopy also permits therapeutic surgical procedures to be performed.

Nursing Interventions: Client education includes an explanation of the procedure. This procedure is most commonly performed in the operating room; thus, appropriate presurgical and anesthesia nursing responsibilities are implemented. Clients are NPO past midnight prior to this procedure. The joint area may be shaved and scrubbed according to protocol.

Description of the Procedure: This procedure is performed with inpatients and outpatients in an arthroscopy room or operating room. The client is positioned according to the joint to be examined. The knee is partially or fully flexed to allow maximum space for insertion of the arthroscope. The entry site is located and prepared. A large bore needle is inserted and the joint space is distended with saline solution. The arthroscope is introduced and the synovium, articular surfaces, and menisci visualized. Before removing the arthroscope, excess saline solution is allowed to drain. The joint is wrapped tightly with an ace bandage or brace. Arthroscopy is completed in less than 1 hour. Visualization results are available immediately.

Evaluating Client Response: Appropriate postanesthesia monitoring is instituted. Vital signs are obtained frequently until stable and the entry site is monitored for signs of bleeding or infection. The ace bandage may be left in place for up to 24 hours. Adequacy of circulation distal to the ace bandage is assessed. Ice may also be applied to reduce swelling. Food and medications are resumed. Analgesics are administered as needed. The examined joint is rested for 1–3 days. Client education about specific joint reconditioning and preventing reoccurring trauma is provided as appropriate. An appointment for removal of the sutures is made as needed. Client and family support in dealing with the results is provided.

BIOPSY

- **Arthrocentesis**
- **Transiliac Bone Biopsy**
- **Muscle Biopsy**
- **Nerve Biopsy**

Many pathophysiologies require biopsy for definitive diagnosis. A specific consent form is required for these procedures.

Nursing Diagnoses for clients undergoing biopsy include:

- Alteration in comfort related to procedure
- Alteration in skin integrity related to procedure
- Anxiety related to diagnostic process
- Knowledge deficit related to procedure

Arthrocentesis (Synovial Fluid Analysis)

Subjective Data: Client complains of pain or altered mobility.

Objective Data: Altered physical exam including swelling, discoloration, limited range of motion or abnormal results from x-ray.

Assessment: Synovial fluid analysis provides data about the pathophysiology of joint symptoms. The results indicate the presence of lupus erythematosis, gout, trauma, bleeding tendencies, infection, or arthritis of the chronic rheumatoid, hemophilus influenza, or septic type. Arthrocentesis may also be performed as part of a contrast study or for therapeutic reasons, such as draining excess synovial fluid or inserting medication.

Normal Values:

Volume: <3.5 ml	Glucose: 70–100 mg/100 ml
Viscosity: high	White Blood Cells: 0–200 μl
Fibrin Clot: absent	Neutrophils: <25%
Mucin Clot: abundant	Protein: 1–3 g/100 ml

Nursing Interventions: Client education includes an explanation of the procedure. Clients may be NPO prior to this procedure. The joint area may be shaved and washed according to protocol. If present during the procedure, the nurse provides emotional support, helps the client maintain a still position, and provides technical assistance.

Description of the Procedure: Arthrocentesis is performed with inpatients and outpatients. The client is positioned with the desired joint fully extended. The entry site is located and the area is prepped. A local anesthetic is administered. A syringe is inserted into the joint and fluid is aspirated. If medication is to be inserted, it is done after fluid has been aspirated. The needle is removed and pressure is applied. This procedure is completed in less than 15 minutes. The results are available following interpretation.

Evaluating Client Response: Postprocedure nursing care includes maintaining pressure on the entry site for several minutes. The client is assessed for bleeding or infection. Some discomfort is to be expected, but bleeding or signs of infection, such as temperature elevation or localized redness are reported to the physician. Food and medications are resumed. The client is instructed to report any delayed increase in soreness, redness or temperature elevation. The examined joint is rested for 24–48 hours. Analgesics are administered as needed.

■ Transiliac Bone Biopsy

Subjective Data: Client complains of pain or changes in mobility.

Objective Data: Altered physical exam or the presence of physiologic fractures or repeated trauma on x-ray.

Assessment: Transiliac bone biopsy provides a measurement of bone mass. Since tetracycline is absorbed by bone tissue and deposited in areas of active mineralization, tetracycline uptake serves as an indicator of the time sequence in bone mineralization. This procedure is used to exclude osteomalacia or osteitis fibrosa in order to establish a diagnosis and treatment for osteoporosis.

Nursing Interventions: Preprocedure nursing responsibilities include an explanation of the procedure. The client's ability to cooperate with the medication regimen is determined. Explicit instructions emphasize the importance of taking the tetracycline as ordered, three times a day for 3 days and then again in the same manner 2 weeks later. Clients are told to take tetracycline 1 hour before or 2 hours after food or antacid intake to prevent any interference with absorption. The client is prepared for postbiopsy discomfort and is made aware that measures can be taken to reduce the discomfort. Activity restrictions after the procedure are discussed. If present during the procedure, the nurse provides emotional support, helps the client maintain a still position and provides technical assistance.

Description of the Procedure: Transiliac bone biopsy is performed with inpatients and outpatients. The client takes tetracycline 250 mg three times daily orally for 3 days. The 3-day course is repeated 2 weeks later. The transiliac bone biopsy is performed within several days of the end of the second course of tetracycline. The biopsy is done in an operating room under strict aseptic conditions. The client receives sedation and local anesthesia. The entry site is located and prepared. A special bone biopsy needle 5–8 mm in diameter is inserted and a bone sample aspirated. After the needle is withdrawn, a pressure dressing is applied. The procedure is completed in less than 15 minutes. The results are available following laboratory analysis and interpretation.

Evaluating Client Response: Following the procedure, the client is monitored for bleeding at the entry site or signs of infection. Local discomfort is expected and may last for several days. An ice pack over the dressing, restricted activity and analgesics are used to reduce discomfort. Unless specifically contraindicated, clients may ambulate later in the day.

■ Muscle Biopsy

Subjective Data: Client complains of pain or changes in mobility.

Objective Data: Findings include altered neuromuscular exam including decreased muscle strength and mass and equivocal results from other testing.

Assessment: The muscle selected for biopsy must be moderately affected by the disease for optimal analysis and interpretation. Muscle biopsy can differentiate myasthenia gravis, muscular dystrophy, inflammatory myositis, infantile hypotonia, Duchenne type of muscular dystrophy, nemaline myopathy, and infantile spinal muscular atrophy. The extent and chronicity of muscle undergoing denervation can be determined. This procedure may or may not be performed in an operating room.

Nursing Interventions: Client education includes an explanation of the procedure and the need to rest the muscle completely following the procedure. If this procedure is being performed in an operating room, appropriate presurgical nursing responsibilities are implemented.

Description of the Procedure: Muscle biopsy is performed with inpatients and outpatients. For needle biopsy, the client is positioned so that the desired muscle is at rest. The entry site is located and prepared. Local anesthesia is administered, specifically avoiding direct injection into the muscle. The needle is inserted, the specimen aspirated, and the needle withdrawn. A bandage or pressure dressing may be applied. The tissue is transported to the lab immediately. The procedure is completed in less than 10 minutes. The results are available following interpretation.

Evaluating Client Response: Following the procedure, the client is monitored for bleeding or hematoma formation at the entry site. Several hours rest are provided for the biopsied muscle, depending on the biopsy procedure used. Children may need slings or restraints to rest the biopsied muscle. Analgesics are administered as needed. With surgical biopsy, sutures may be used and these are removed in 7–10 days. Client and family support in dealing with the results is provided as needed.

■ Nerve Biopsy

Subjective Data: Client complains of pain, tingling, and other peripheral sensory changes.

Objective Data: Altered neurologic exam including altered dermatomes and equivocal results from other testing.

Assessment: Nerve biopsy is performed to establish an accurate diagnosis of peripheral neuropathy. The extent of damage to myelinated and unmyelinated nerve fibers or axons can be determined, as can myelin damage or selective injury to nerve fibers of a specific diameter. The sural nerve, which runs down the back of the leg from just above the knee to the end of the foot, is the most common site for nerve biopsy. The client usually experiences some degree of temporary sensory loss, but long-term effects or complications are not common.

Nursing Interventions: Client education includes an explanation of the procedure and the need for rest after the procedure. The usually temporary nature of postprocedure sensory loss is discussed. If present during the procedure, the nurse provides emotional support, helps the client maintain a still position, and provides technical assistance.

Description of the Procedure: Nerve biopsy by needle aspiration is performed on inpatients and outpatients. For needle biopsy, the client is positioned so the desired nerve can be easily reached. The entry site is located and prepared. Local anesthesia is administered. A needle is inserted and when the nerve is located, a small specimen is aspirated and the needle withdrawn. A bandage may be applied. The tissue is transported to the lab immediately. The procedure is completed in less than 10 minutes. The results are available following interpretation.

Evaluating Client Response: Following the procedure, the client is monitored for bleeding or hematoma formation at the entry site. The biopsied nerve is rested for several hours. Analgesics are administered as needed. Client and family reassurance regarding the expected temporary sensory loss is provided as needed.

SPINAL PUNCTURE

- **Lumbar Puncture and Manometric Test**
- **Spinal Dynamics**
- **Lateral Cervical Puncture**
- **Cisternal Puncture**
- **Subdural Puncture**

For clients with impaired mobility, spinal puncture may be performed as part of a contrast study or to measure spinal dynamics. Although lumbar puncture is the most common procedure, other puncture sites are used. Spinal dynamics are performed to obtain pressure readings and cerebrospinal fluid for laboratory analysis. A specific consent form is required for these procedures.

Nursing Diagnoses for clients undergoing spinal puncture include:

- Alteration in comfort related to procedure
- Anxiety related to procedure
- Knowledge deficit related to diagnostic process
- Potential for infection related to procedure

■ Lumbar Puncture (LP, Spinal Tap) and Manometric Test

Subjective Data: Client complains of headache, pain, or altered neurologic functioning.

Objective Data: Altered neurologic exam, including changes in gait, speech, vision, or mental status exam, and abnormal data from other tests such as x-ray, scintigraphy, CT, or MR.

Assessment: Lumbar puncture is performed to measure CSF pressure, obtain CSF for laboratory analysis, perform spinal dynamics, or insert a contrast medium for radiographic visualization of the nervous system. Manometric test refers to the measuring of pressures, especially the opening pressure. LPs are also done for therapeutic reasons including removing blood or pus from the subarachnoid space, injecting drugs and sera, reducing intracranial pressure, or producing spinal anesthesia. Diagnostic LPs are contraindicated in clients with suspected intracranial tumor, with clinical evidence of increased intracranial pressure, or with infection of skin or bone at the puncture site.

Normal Values for Cerebrospinal Fluid:

Pressure: 60–180 mm H_2O.
Visual Inspection: clear, odorless, colorless.
Red Blood Cells: none.
White Blood Cells: 0–5 agranulocytes/cubic mm.
Microorganisms: none.
Protein: 15–45 mg/100 ml lumbar sample.
15–25 mg/100 ml cisternal sample.
5–15 mg/100 ml ventricular sample.
Chloride: 118–132 mEq/100 ml.
Glutamine: 6–20 mg/100 ml.
Glucose: 60–80% of serum level or 40–80 mg/100 ml.
Lactic Acid: 20–28 mg/100 ml.
LDH: 10% of serum level or 6–15 U.
Urea: 7–15 mg/100 ml.

Nursing Interventions: Client education includes an explanation of the procedure. The importance of achieving and maintaining the correct position is emphasized. Although positioning is essential to allow safe entry into the subarachnoid space, pressure measurements are inaccurate if the child is crying and fighting. Child management techniques, restraints, and sedation are used to help the child cooperate. Postprocedure monitoring is discussed and the "routineness" emphasized so that the client does not misinterpret the frequent nursing actions. The client is asked to empty bowel and bladder prior to the procedure. The client may receive a sedative 30 minutes prior to the procedure with appropriate safety precautions being implemented. If present during the procedure, the nurse provides emotional support, helps the client maintain a still position, and provides technical assistance.

Description of the Procedure: LPs are usually performed with inpatients. Vital signs and a baseline neurologic assessment are obtained. Privacy is provided. If an opening pressure is not being obtained, the client may sit and lean over a table. Otherwise, the client lies at the edge of the bed or examining table and is assisted into a fetal position, knees-to-chest, head and shoulders bent over, and hands grasped below the knees. A small pillow may be placed under the head and a large pillow between the knees. This position provides maximal space at the entry site, the interspace between the 3rd and 4th lumbar vertebrae in line with the iliac crest. The entry site may be lower in the spinal canal as the cord extends further in infants and young children. The client is draped and the entry site is located and prepared. Local anesthesia is administered until a wheal is formed. A stylet is inserted through the wheal until fluid drips out, indicating entry into the subarachnoid space. A stopcock and manometer are attached and the opening pressure reading is obtained. The client may be allowed to relax the legs to reduce pressure on the abdomen. Using the stopcock, 8–10 ml of CSF are allowed to drip into 3–4 different test tubes. To avoid potential contamination and resulting error in interpretation, the first test tube is not used for CSF culture. The closing pressure is obtained and the stylet is removed. A bandage is applied to the entry site. The procedure is completed in less than 10 minutes. The results are available following interpretation.

Evaluating Client Response: Following the procedure, the client's vital signs and neurologic status are monitored every 15 minutes the first hour, every 30 minutes the second hour, every hour thereafter until stable, and then every 4 hours prn. Adverse neurologic signs include changes in pupillary dilation, level of consciousness or motor function, or nuchal rigidity. Bleeding or leakage at the entry site are also reported immediately. The client may be required to stay flat in bed for 4–12 hours. The head of the bed may be elevated 15 degrees for meals. Headaches are common sequellae and may be somewhat relieved by having the client lie flat in bed. Pain medication is administered as needed. Temperature is monitored because an increase, with or without chills, may be associated with nuchal rigidity from meningeal irritation. Increased fluid intake to at least 3000 ml in 24 hours enhances CSF fluid replacement and may reduce headaches. Client and family support in dealing with the results is provided.

■ Spinal Dynamics (Queckenstedt Test)

Subjective Data: Client complains of headache, pain, or altered neurologic functioning.

Objective Data: Altered neurologic exam including changes in mental status, vision, speech, or gait, and abnormal results from other tests such as x-ray, scintigraphy, CT, or MR.

Assessment: This procedure is used to determine if spinal cord compression is present and if so, if it is complete or partial. The Queckenstedt test determines variations in CSF pressure in response to timed bilateral compression of the jugular veins. It is contraindicated in the presence of increased intracranial pressure, hemorrhage, or suspected CNS tumor. Normal results include a rise in pressure of at least 100 mm from the baseline and a return to baseline within 30 seconds.

Nursing Interventions: Client education includes an explanation of the procedure. Positioning is explained. Although positioning is essential to allow safe entry into the subarachnoid space, pressure measurements are inaccurate if the child is crying and fighting. Restraints, sedation, and child management techniques are used to help the child cooperate. The role of breath holding during the initial phase is discussed, as is application of pressure during the second phase. The client is prepared to experience sensations of fullness, local constriction, and facial warmth. The transitory nature of these sensations is emphasized. Postprocedure monitoring and its "routineness" are discussed so that the client does not misinterpret the frequent nursing actions. The client is prepared for post-procedure bed rest, increased fluid intake, and the availability of analgesia. Client support for the diagnostic process is provided. If present during the procedure, the nurse provides emotional support, helps the client maintain a still position, and provides technical assistance.

Description of the Procedure: This procedure is performed with inpatients. In infants and young children the entry site may be lower in the spinal canal as the cord extends further. A lumbar puncture with the client in the lateral recumbent position is performed as previously described to the point at which the stylet is to be connected. For this procedure, the stylet is connected to a calibrated manometer. The "initial pressure" reading is taken before any fluid is removed. The client's position is adjusted and the client made comfortable in the left lateral position with legs relaxed and straight. The head and neck are supported in proper alignment. The client takes a deep breath, holds it, and strains as if for a bowel movement for a total of 10 seconds. A pressure reading is obtained and the client relaxes. Pressure readings are repeated every 5 seconds until they return to normal, in order to determine patency of the stylet and the ability of the client to cooperate. This procedure is repeated as needed until a satisfactory response is attained from the manometer and client. As the client relaxes, the next step is explained. The client is told not to cough or suspend respirations. Pressure is applied, either manually or with a sphygmomanometer inflated to 40 mm Hg, for 10 seconds to both jugular veins. The pressure is released and measurements are obtained every 5 seconds until they return to baseline. The stylet is withdrawn and a bandage placed over the entry site. This procedure is completed in less than 1 hour. The results are available immediately.

Evaluating Client Response: Following the procedure, the client's vital signs and neurologic status are monitored every 15 minutes the first hour, every 30 minutes the second hour, every hour until stable, and then every 4 hours prn. Adverse neurologic signs include change in pupillary dilation, level of consciousness or motor function, and nuchal rigidity. Bleeding or leakage from the entry site are also reported immediately. The client may be required to stay flat in bed. The head of the bed may be elevated 15 degrees for meals. Headaches are common sequellae and may be somewhat relieved by having the client lie flat in bed. Pain medication is administered as needed. Temperature is monitored because an increase, with or without chills, may be associated with nuchal rigidity from meningeal irritation. Increased fluid intake to at least 3000 ml in 24 hours enhances CSF fluid replacement and may help to reduce headaches. Client and family support in dealing with the results is provided.

■ Lateral Cervical Puncture

Subjective Data: Client complains of headache, pain, or altered neurologic functioning.

Objective Data: Altered neurologic exam, including changes in gait, speech, vision, or mental status exam, and abnormal data from other tests such as x-ray, scintigraphy, CT, or MR.

Assessment: For lateral cervical puncture, the entry site is the C1–C2 interspace. This procedure is performed on clients in whom a lumbar puncture is contraindicated, such as clients with a superficial infection, acute traumatic damage to the lumbar area, gross obesity, arachnoiditis, spinal column bony deformity, or those unable to flex the neck to avoid the complications of cisternal puncture.

Nursing Interventions: Client education includes an explanation of the procedure. The required position is explained and the client is prepared to experience a "pop" as the stylet is inserted. Pressure measurements are inaccurate if the child is crying and fighting. Child management techniques, restraints, and sedation are used to help the child cooperate. Postprocedure monitoring and its "routineness" are discussed so that the client does not misinterpret the frequent nursing actions. The client is prepared for bed rest, an increased fluid intake, the potential for headache, and the availability of analgesic relief. Client support for the diagnostic process is provided. The client is asked to empty bowel and bladder prior to the procedure. The client may receive a sedative 30 minutes prior to the procedure and if so, appropriate nursing actions regarding safety are implemented. If present during the procedure, the nurse provides emotional support, helps the client maintain a still position, and provides technical assistance.

Description of the Procedure: This procedure is performed with inpatients. Vital signs and a neurologic assessment are obtained for a baseline. Privacy is assured. The client is prone without a pillow and the neck extended as straight as possible. The client is told not to cough or breathe abnormally. The entry site, 1 cm caudal and 1 cm posterior to the landmark on the cervical spine, is located and prepared. Local anesthesia is administered until a wheal is formed. The stylet is inserted through the wheal until fluid drips out. As the tissue planes are entered, the client feels a "pop." A stopcock and manometer are attached and the opening pressure reading is obtained. Using the stopcock, 8–10 ml of CSF are allowed to drip into 3–4 different test tubes. To avoid potential contamination and resulting error in interpretation, the first test tube is not used for CSF culture. The closing pressure is obtained and the stylet is removed. A bandage is applied to the entry site. The procedure is completed in less than 10 minutes. The results are available following analysis and interpretation.

Evaluating Client Response: Following the procedure, the client's vital signs and neurologic status are monitored every 15 minutes the first hour, every 30 minutes the second hour, every hour until stable, and then every 4 hours prn. Adverse neurologic signs include changes in pupillary dilation, level of consciousness or motor function, nuchal rigidity, and bleeding or leaking from the entry site, and are reported to the physician immediately. The client lies flat for 4–6 hours, but may have a small pillow if requested. The client's neck is supported during turning. Headaches are common sequellae and may be somewhat relieved by having the client lie flat in bed. Pain medication is administered as ordered. Temperature is monitored because an increase, with or without chills, may be associated with nuchal rigidity from meningeal irritation. Increased fluid intake to at least 3000 ml in 24 hours enhances CSF fluid replacement and may help reduce headaches. Client and family support in dealing with the results is provided.

■ Cisternal Puncture

Subjective Data: Client complains of headache, pain, or altered neuromuscular functioning.

Objective Data: Altered neurologic exam, including changes in gait, speech, vision, or mental status exam, and abnormal data from other tests such as x-ray, scintigraphy, CT, or MR.

Assessment: Cisternal puncture provides less risk for the client. It is performed to remove CSF on outpatients, to insert contrast media during myelography and encephalography, and may be done simultaneously with lumbar puncture to demonstrate a subarachnoid block.

Nursing Interventions: Client education includes an explanation of the procedure. The importance of client cooperation in achieving and maintaining the desired position is explained. Cisternal puncture is usually part of a radiologic procedure in children. Restraints, sedation, and child management techniques may be needed to help the child cooperate. Postprocedure monitoring is discussed. The client is asked to empty bowel and bladder. If present during the procedure, the nurse provides emotional support, helps the client maintain a still position, and provides technical assistance.

Description of the Procedure: Cisternal puncture is performed with inpatients and outpatients. Vital signs and a neurologic assessment are obtained for a baseline. Privacy is assured. The client is positioned prone on the examining table. The entry site, in a median line below the occipital bone, is located and prepared. Local anesthesia may or may not be used. The stylet is inserted approximately 5 cm until fluid drips out, indicating entry into the cisterna magna. CSF fluid is removed and/or a contrast medium inserted depending on client need. The stylet is removed. A bandage is applied to the entry site. This procedure is completed in less than 10 minutes; however, more time is required for radiologic follow-up. The results are available following analysis and interpretation.

Evaluating Client Response: Postprocedure client evaluation includes assessing the client for cyanosis, dyspnea, or apnea. Level of consciousness, vital signs, and bleeding from the entry site are monitored every 15 minutes the first hour, every 30 minutes the second hour, and every hour until stable. The client may then be discharged. Clients are advised against overexertion for 24 hours. If CSF fluid has been removed, an increased fluid intake is encouraged.

■ Subdural Puncture (Ventricular Tap)

Subjective Data: Infants may appear uncomfortable, cranky, and irritable. Adults may complain of mental status changes.

Objective Data: Altered neurologic exam including changes in mental status, vision, speech, or gait and/or altered data from other testing such as x-ray, scintigraphy, CT, or MR.

Assessment: This procedure is performed on infants and children whose cranial suture lines are open. It is used to identify hydrocephalus, subdural effusion, subdural or ventricular hemorrhage, or bacteria in the subdural or ventricular spaces. It may also be performed to localize a tumor when encephalography is contraindicated or for therapeutic purposes, such as medication instillation or relief of intracranial pressure. It is also performed on adults following craniotomy or craniectomy to remove fluid quickly.

Nursing Interventions: Education of clients or the parents includes an explanation of the procedure and the need to shave the scalp. Routine postprocedure monitoring and bed rest are discussed. If the subdural tap is to be an operative procedure, the appropriate nursing actions are implemented. If present during the procedure, the nurse provides emotional support, helps the client maintain a still position, and provides technical assistance.

Description of the Procedure: Subdural taps are performed with inpatients. The anterior two-thirds of the scalp is shaved. The child is supine with the head immobilized and facing forward. Baseline vital signs and neurologic assessment are obtained. The entry site, either at the junction of the anterior fontanel and coronal suture or a few millimeters away from the fontanel in the suture line, is located and prepared. The client is draped. Local anesthesia is administered. A short lumbar puncture needle is inserted until fluid drips out or until the dura mater is punctured. CSF is allowed to flow into 3–4 different test tubes. Usually, subdural taps are performed bilaterally. A new needle is used for the second tap. If a contrast medium is being inserted, it is first diluted with removed CSF. Less than 30 ml of CSF is removed to prevent sudden intracranial decompression and shock. The needle is removed and a dressing is applied to the entry site. The procedure is completed in less than 10 minutes; however, more time is required for radiologic testing. The results are available following analysis and interpretation.

Evaluating Client Response: Following the procedure, the client is assessed for changes in the level of consciousness or skin color and leakage or bleeding from the entry site. Vital signs are monitored every 30 minutes until stable and then every 4 hours prn. Adverse neurologic signs include changes in pupillary dilation, level of consciousness or motor function, bleeding or leaking at the entry site, and are reported to the physician immediately. The client is kept flat in bed for 24 hours. Support for client and family in dealing with the results is provided.

CONTRAST STUDIES

- Arthrography
- Digital Subtraction Angiography
- Carotid Angiography
- Myelography
- Air Encephalography

Since impaired mobility can result from many different pathophysiologies, many different contrast studies are used. Contrast media are inserted into the joints, the arterial system, and the spinal column. The degree of invasiveness, and therefore impact on the client, correlates with the entry site and/or the area being studied. A specific informed consent is required for these procedures.

Nursing Diagnoses for clients undergoing contrast studies include:

- Alteration in comfort related to procedure
- Anxiety related to procedure
- Knowledge deficit related to diagnostic process
- Potential for infection related to procedure
- Potential for injury: allergic reaction related to procedure

Arthrography

Subjective Data: Client complains of pain and changes in joint motion.

Objective Data: Altered physical findings including swelling, discoloration, dislocation, or limited range of motion.

Assessment: Arthrography is used to examine the synovial cavity for pathology of the joint capsule, cartilage, and supporting ligaments. Arthrograms are most frequently used for the knees, shoulders, and hips. Arthrography is contraindicated in the presence of acute infection.

Nursing Interventions: Client education includes an explanation of the procedure. The need to cooperate with joint motion is emphasized. Children may require additional assistance during this procedure. Clients are told that some discomfort may occur and that analgesics and ice are available to reduce the discomfort. A client history specific for prior allergic response to iodine or radiopaque media is obtained. The client wears a hospital gown, removes all jewelry and prostheses, and voids prior to the procedure.

Description of the Procedure. This procedure is performed with inpatients and outpatients. The client goes to an x-ray room. The entry site into the joint is located and prepared. Local anesthesia is administered. A needle is inserted into the joint space and the contrast medium is instilled. Air may also be inserted. Fluoroscopy and serial radiographs are obtained as the joint is put through its full range of motion. Then the needle is withdrawn. This procedure is completed in 1–2 hours. Preliminary results may be available immediately, but final interpretation follows detailed viewing of the films.

Evaluating Client Response: Following the procedure, the client is evaluated for bleeding or signs of infection at the insertion site. Analgesics and ice may help reduce client discomfort. Client and family support is provided in dealing with the results.

■ Digital Subtraction Angiography (DSA)

Subjective Data: Client complains of pain, headache, changes in vision and hearing, numbness, or other changes in neurologic functions.

Objective Data: Altered physical findings including carotid bruits and abnormal results from other diagnostic tests, e.g., ocular plethysmography and doppler ultrasonography.

Assessment: This procedure uses an image-enhancement system, known as "mask mode subtraction," to amplify low-concentration intravascular iodine signals. The results provide data about arterial blood flow to the brain and are used to evaluate clients with cervicocerebral atherosclerotic disease. Two contrast medium injection techniques are in use. IV DSA involves a rapid injection of 150–200 ml of contrast material into the brachial vein or superior vena cava. This technique is considered safer. IA DSA provides a clearer image but requires threading a catheter into the aortic arch and injecting a smaller volume of contrast material. The need for complete absence of motion makes this procedure unsuitable for infants and young children unless general anesthesia is used.

Nursing Interventions: Client education includes an explanation of the procedure. The ability of the client to lie perfectly still and not swallow has a major impact on the success of this procedure and this is explained to the client. Postprocedure monitoring is discussed. A client history specific for allergy to iodine and previous reaction to contrast media is obtained. For IV DSA, adequacy of kidney function is determined as the client receives 150–250 ml of contrast medium solution over 30–60 minutes. For IA DSA, adequacy of clotting status is determined in order to prevent postprocedure complications. Adjustment in anticoagulant therapy may be needed. Clients may be NPO for 2–6 hours before the procedure. The client wears a hospital gown, removes all jewelry and prostheses, and voids prior to the procedure.

Description of the Procedure: DSA is performed with inpatients and outpatients. The client reclines and is positioned relative to the fluoroscopic camera. The mask is recorded and stored by computer. The entry site is prepared. The contrast medium is administered by one of the methods discussed above and the second image is obtained. Respiratory or other movement including swallowing may render the images unsatisfactory. If this occurs, another mask can be obtained after the contrast medium has left the region. This procedure is completed in approximately 1 hour. Results are available following interpretation.

Evaluating Client Response: Following the procedure, the client is monitored for bleeding at the entry site. Distal pulses and blood pressure are monitored every 15 minutes the first hour, every 30 minutes the next 2 hours, and every 4 hours thereafter prn. Neurologic status is assessed frequently and adverse changes reported immediately. Food and medications are resumed. Fluid intake is increased to approximately 2 liters to aid in excretion of the contrast medium. If a catheter was threaded into the aortic arch, postprocedure care follows the guidelines for postangiography nursing care. Outpatients are instructed to check for postprocedure bleeding and to return if any bleeding is noted. Outpatients should not drive themselves home. Client and family support in dealing with the results is provided.

■ Carotid Angiography (Cerebral Arteriography)

Subjective Data: Client complains of pain, headache, changes in vision and hearing, and other changes in neurologic function.

Objective Data: Bruits, altered neurologic exam including vision, speech, gait, or mental status, and altered data from other tests, e.g., x-ray, scintigraphy, CT, or MR.

Assessment: This procedure is the definitive diagnostic method for assessing the position, size, placement, and disruption of cerebral circulation. Cerebral angiography demonstrates subarachnoid hemorrhage, vessel occlusion or obstruction, vascular lesions, arteriovenous malformation, aneurysm, and space-occupying lesions. The earlier angiography is performed in terms of onset of symptoms, the more definitive it is for embolism. The presence of arterial spasm can also be assessed. The catheter is inserted via the brachial or femoral artery. Due to the risk inherent in entering an artery, other procedures precede angiography in the diagnostic process.

Nursing Interventions: Client education includes an explanation of the procedure and the need to remain still. The ability of the child to cooperate and the need for additional sedation and/or restraint is determined. Clients are told that injection of the contrast medium may cause an unpleasant feeling. Clients are told in advance of the routine postprocedure monitoring and bed rest. A client history specific for prior allergic response to iodine or radiopaque media is obtained. Adequacy of clotting status is determined. Anticoagulant therapy is temporarily interrupted. Clients are well-hydrated 24–48 hours prior to this procedure but are NPO for 6 hours before it begins. The client receives sedation and appropriate nursing actions are implemented. The client wears a hospital gown and removes all jewelry and prostheses.

Description of the Procedure: This procedure is usually performed with inpatients. Baseline vital signs and neurologic assessment are obtained. In an x-ray room, the entry site is located and prepared. Local anesthesia is administered and the entry site draped. The client is instructed not to move until visualization is complete. A catheter is inserted into the femoral artery and via fluoroscopy is threaded in retrograde fashion through the aorta into the arch and the cerebral vessels. The contrast medium is inserted through the catheter and serial timed radiographs are obtained. The catheter is withdrawn and a dressing is applied to the entry site. Many clients report discomfort during this procedure. This procedure is completed in approximately 60 minutes. Preliminary results may be available immediately, but final interpretation follows detailed viewing of the films.

Evaluating Client Response: Following the procedure, direct pressure is applied to the entry site and the client lies supine with the entry site immobilized for 2–6 hours. The client is evaluated for adverse neurologic signs such as hemiparesis, hemiplegia, aphasia, or decreased level of consciousness. The insertion site and pulses, skin color, and temperature distal to the insertion site are monitored for signs of bleeding. Vital signs and neurologic assessment are obtained every 15 minutes the first hour, every 30 minutes the next 2 hours, and every hour thereafter until stable. Food and medications are resumed. Fluid intake is encouraged to promote excretion of the contrast medium. Analgesics are administered as needed. Client and family support is provided in dealing with the results.

■ Myelography

Subjective Data: Client complains of pain or changes in neuromuscular function.

Objective Data: Altered neuromuscular exam including changes in reflexes and gait and abnormal data from other tests such as x-ray, CT, or MR.

Assessment: Myelograms are used to visualize the subarachnoid space in order to detect abnormalities of the spinal cord or vertebrae and locate obstruction in the flow of CSF in the vertebral subarachnoid space. Myelograms are performed on clients with suspected herniated, ruptured or degenerative intervertebral disc disorder, neoplasm, or abscess. Two different contrast media are in use. Pantopaque, iodophenylundecylic acid, is an oil-based iodine compound requiring considerable tilting of the table and must be removed before completion of the study. Ampaque, metrizamide, is a water-based, noniodine compound that is excreted in the urine within 72 hours. Ampaque exacerbates seizure activity. Air is occasionally used as the contrast medium.

Nursing Interventions: Client education includes an explanation of the procedure and the importance of proper positioning. The ability of the child to cooperate and the need for additional sedation or restraint is determined. The client is prepared for the tilting of the table and some discomfort during the procedure. Postprocedure monitoring and bed rest are discussed. A client history specific for allergy to iodine or previous reaction to contrast media is obtained. Clients are NPO for 4 hours prior to the procedure. The client may be premedicated with narcotics and/or atropine to promote relaxation and drowsiness. Client safety measures are implemented. The client removes all jewelry and prostheses, wears a hospital gown, and voids prior to the procedure.

Description of the Procedure: This procedure is performed with inpatients. The client is taken to the radiology room, placed on a tilt table and assumes a fetal position. The puncture site, usually lumbar but occasionally cervical, is located and prepared. A needle is inserted and 10–15 ml of CSF removed. The contrast medium, either Pantopaque or Ampaque, is inserted. Fluoroscopy and serial timed radiographs of the subarachnoid space are obtained. The table may be tilted for different views. If Pantopaque is the contrast medium used, it is aspirated. Clients may complain of pain during aspiration, due to pressure on a nerve root, which may be eased by rotating the needle. Following completion of the procedure, the needle is withdrawn and a bandage applied. This procedure may require several hours to complete. Preliminary results may be available immediately, but definitive interpretation follows detailed viewing.

Evaluating Client Response: Following the procedure, the client's neurologic status and vital signs are monitored every 30 minutes until stable and then every 2 hours for 24 hours. The entry site is checked for bleeding or leaking. The client's position, which is intended to prevent or reduce postmyelogram headache, is dependent on the contrast medium used. If Pantopaque was used, the client is flat in bed for 6–24 hours. If Ampaque was used, the client is in semifowlers position at 15–30 degrees for 8 hours. Being flat can precipitate seizures in these clients. If air was the contrast medium, the client lies with head lower than body. Food and medications are resumed. Analgesics are administered as needed for headache. Clients are encouraged to drink at least 2500 ml over 24 hours and intake and output are recorded. Clients may need to be assessed for bladder distension and urinary retention. The client requires assistance the first few times he or she stands. Client and family support in dealing with the results is provided.

■ Air Encephalography (Pneumoencephalography, Ventriculography)

These highly invasive procedures were used to examine the ventricles and the subarachnoid space. Risk and discomfort during and after the procedure are high. These procedures are rarely performed today because the newer diagnostic imaging techniques are more accurate. They have been replaced by computed tomography, scintigraphy, and magnetic resonance imaging.

8

Clients with Alterations in Sensory Input

Clients develop alterations in sensory input from many different pathophysiologies and undergo a wide variety of diagnostic procedures. The focus of nursing care for both the disease process and the diagnostic process is communication. The impact of sensory deficits on the individual, the family and society can be enormous. Nevertheless, millions of people cope daily with these problems and lead fulfilling lives. Many devices exist to help clients increase sensory input and a large portion of our society depends on visual and/or hearing aids. For clients with impaired sensory perception, diagnostic testing may be a repetitive event in their lives. Some diagnostic procedures are performed with the client first using and then not using a sensory aid. Nursing diagnoses during the diagnostic process include the psychosocial effects of sensory deprivation as well as the pathophysiologic concerns.

Physical examination is the first step in the diagnostic process for clients with alterations in sensory input. A family history, past medical history, and history of the present illness are obtained. Because impairment in sensory perception may be insidious in onset and gradual in progression, clients may have made adaptations without realizing it. Thus, detailed questioning of the client is mandated in assessing changes in sensory perception.

TESTS FOR SENSORY ACUITY

- **Vision Testing**
- **Tuning Fork Tests**
- **Audiology Tests**

Testing of both visual and hearing acuity may be part of a routine health screening or may be part of a specific diagnostic procedure that determines which corrective measures will benefit the client. In testing sensory input, client cooperation is essential to the accuracy of the results. No specific consent form is required.

Nursing Diagnoses for clients undergoing testing of sensory acuity include:

- Anxiety related to procedure
- Knowledge deficit related to diagnostic process

Vision Tests

Subjective Data: Client complains of changes in vision.

Objective Data: This procedure is usually the first diagnostic procedure performed.

Assessment: Vision testing is performed with people of all ages. As a screening mechanism, minimal equipment is needed, allowing these tests to be performed in a variety of settings.

Nursing Interventions: Client education includes an explanation of the procedure and the importance of client cooperation. The ability of the child to participate is determined. Instructions for children can be made to seem like games.

Description of the Procedure: Vision testing is performed with inpatients and outpatients. The client is placed in a comfortable position. Most of these tests are conducted under normal illumination. The test is explained and the client is asked to respond to what is seen. Visual acuity testing takes from 5–60 minutes and may include one or more tests. Consideration is given to the ability of the client to concentrate for prolonged periods of time and to the potential for eye fatigue if the client is undergoing many tests. The results are available immediately.

Letter Chart, Snellen Eye Test, BVAT (Mentor) Microprocessor: These tests measure visual acuity. Visual acuity is stated in terms of a ratio of the distance at which the client sees to the distance at which the client should see. These tests measure the distance at which the client can see clearly. Each eye is tested individually as the other eye is shielded. The microprocessor uses an E of different sizes. The client operates a hand-held response box. Charts with different objects are used to test children who are too young or developmentally unable to accurately read the alphabet.

Color Plates: These are used to assess color perception. Each plate is covered with different colored dots. The dots of one color form a design, number, or object, and the client identifies the design seen on each plate. Color plates for testing children contain common objects, i.e., a ball, a wagon, etc.

Automated Clinical Refractor: These are used to determine visual acuity in clients with opacities. They are used to separate retinal and neurologic factors from optical limiting factors. This test also provides predictive data on the degree of improvement in visual acuity that can be expected from cataract surgery. The client is required to remain still and look straight ahead. With objective instruments, the operator focuses the light on the retina and a machine measures the astigmatism. With subjective refractors, the client looks into the machine and turns a knob to focus on and answer questions about various targets. Generally, children 6 years of age or younger need objective refraction, whereas 7–8 year olds can use the subjective refractors reliably. Cycoplegic agents are usually used for refraction in young children.

Worth 4-Dot Test, Red Filter Test, and Lancaster Projector Tests: These tests are used to determine ocular mobility and strabismus by testing for fusion, suppression, and anomalous retinal correspondence. For the Worth 4-dot test, a red filter is placed in front of one eye and a green filter in front of the other. The client is exposed to two green lights, one red light, and one white light. Normally, a client sees white light through both filters, and colored lights only through the same color filter. The red filter test uses only red filters. The Lancaster projector uses a machine to project the lights and has controls for the client to superimpose the targets.

Bagoline Striated Glasses Test: The client wears glasses with a faint reference line on each lens. Adjustment of the lens is made to determine the diagnosis.

Major Amblyscope Test: This test is used to investigate fusion. The client looks into the tubes of the amblyscope at two pictures that are identical except for one or two details. Normally, a client can identify the differences in detail.

Afterimage Test: This test is used with older children with suspected strabismus. A long electric filament is used; it is approximately 30 cm long with the central 4 cm blocked out. The client is asked to focus on the center gap. The filament is shown vertically to the right eye for 15 seconds while the left eye is shielded, and then horizontally to the left eye while the right eye is shielded. Positive afterimages are seen with either eye closed or in the dark, whereas negative afterimages are best brought out in the dark.

Vectorgraphic Test for Suppression: This test uses the A–O Vectorgraphic Project-O-Chart Slide (by American Optical Company). Each character on the slide has self-contained illumination at a different angle. Normally, all six letters are read without hesitation, although only two letters are seen by the right eye, two letters only by the left eye, and two letters by both eyes.

Evaluating Client Response: If the client's eyes have been dilated, the need for safe transportation is assessed. The client is told how long the effects of eye drops may last.

■ Tuning Fork Tests

Subjective Data: Client complains of changes in hearing.

Objective Data: These are usually the first diagnostic procedures performed.

Assessment: Tuning fork tests are used as preliminary screening techniques for hearing acuity. Most frequently, 512 cycles/second, Hertz, tuning forks are used.

Nursing Interventions: Client preparation includes an explanation of the procedure.

Description of the Procedure: Since minimal equipment is required, these tests can be performed anywhere. The client is placed in a comfortable position and the tests conducted. The tests take less than 10 minutes. The results are available immediately.

Weber Test: This test is for lateralization and is suggestive of conductive or sensorineural problems. The tuning fork is rapped and placed on the skull in the midline. Normally, the client hears the sound equally in both ears.

Renne Test: This test compares air conduction (AC) to bone conduction (BC). The tuning fork is rapped and first placed on the mastoid bone as near as possible to the pinna without touching it. The tuning fork is then moved and held 2 inches away from and lateral to the ear canal. Normally, AC is greater than BC.

Modified Schwabach Test: This involves placing the rapped tuning fork on the mastoid bone and asking the client to state when the sound is no longer heard. Normally, the length of time is bilaterally equal.

Evaluating Client Response: The results are explained to the client.

■ Audiology Tests (Audiogram, Impedance Audiometry)

Subjective Data: Client complains of changes in hearing or tinnitus.

Objective Data: Altered findings from tuning fork testing.

Assessment: Audiology testing provides quantitative measurement of the client's hearing. Standard basic audiograms include both Air and Bone Pure Tone tests, the Speech Reception test and the Speech Discrimination test. Hearing tests are used for routine screenings and for specific diagnostic assessment. The results of audiologic tests are used to diagnose hearing loss and to determine the most effective form of treatment. If a hearing aid is recommended, test results are used to determine the most effective device for each client. Client cooperation is essential for accurate results. Testing may include repeating a stimulus to determine client reliability in responding.

Diagnostic audiology uses a qualitative test to determine the presence and location of pathology in the auditory system. The location of a lesion, in the middle ear, coclea, 8th cranial nerve, or central auditory system, is determined. The pattern of results from several tests is used to formulate a diagnosis. A wide variety of tests are used. Difficult speech audiometry, the tone decay test, and impedance audiometry are included here. The auditory brain stem response test records electrical activity generated by the 8th cranial nerve stimulation and is discussed in Measurement of Electrical Activity in Chapter 7.

Nursing Interventions: Client education includes an explanation of the procedure and the importance of client cooperation. The ability of the child to reliably cooperate during testing is determined. Children may drop balls instead of raising a finger to signal. Rewards, such as moving puppets, may be used to maintain the child's interest. Impedance audiometry is particularly well-suited for young children, since it requires little cooperation, provides objective results, and is quick and easy to administer.

Description of the Procedure: Audiology tests are performed with inpatients and outpatients. The client goes to the audiology room, a shielded, sound-proof room connected by a window to the room where the examiner sits. The client wears one or two sets of headphones for part or all of the testing. The client is instructed before each test as to how to respond. Testing time varies and is completed in 10–45 minutes. The results are available immediately.

Pure Tone Air Conduction and Pure Tone Bone Conduction Tests: These tests are performed to determine the level, in decibels, at which a client can hear a pure tone, stated in terms of frequency of cycles per second, or "hertz." The client signals as soon as a tone is heard. Normally, frequencies of 125–8000 Hz are heard at 25 or less decibels.

Speech Reception Test (SRT): The client is asked to repeat a 36-word list of spondee words, words of two syllables with equal emphasis on both syllables, such as airplane, hotdog, etc. The threshhold level is that level at which the client can accurately repeat approximately 50% of the words.

Speech Discrimination Test (SD): The client is asked to repeat a list of 50 monosyllabic familiar words that are considered equally difficult to understand and are phonetically balanced to represent the frequency of occurrence in everyday English.

Difficult Speech Audiometry: The performance intensity (PI) function is obtained by using phonetically balanced (PB) monosyllabic words. Testing continues beyond the threshhold plateau at which the client can hear.

Tone Decay Test (ART, Impedance Audiometry): This test measures acoustic impedance at the tympanic membrane as the stapedius muscle contracts in response to a loud stimulus. The electroacoustic impedance meter, a sound and pressure measuring device, is used. A probe seals the external auditory canal. Within the probe are three areas. One produces a stimulus, the second measures the intensity of the stimulus with a microphone, and the third area connects to a manometer that measures pressure changes within the canal. The test is not uncomfortable for the client.

Evaluating Client Response: The results are explained to the client.

DIRECT VISUALIZATION

- ■ Ophthalmoscopy
- ■ Gonioscopy

Direct visualization of the eye is unique in that it is not an invasive procedure. Thus, highly informative diagnostic data are obtained at minimal client risk. These procedures may be part of a routine screening program or may be performed for a specific diagnostic purpose. A fundus camera may be used to record the findings. A specific consent form is not required.

Nursing Diagnoses for clients undergoing direct visualization of the eye include:

- ▶ Anxiety related to procedure
- ▶ Temporary altered sensory input related to procedure
- ▶ Knowledge deficit related to diagnostic process

■ Ophthalmoscopy

Subjective Data: Client complains of blurred vision, loss of vision, changes in visual clarity of field, or pain.

Objective Data: Routine screening or altered findings on visual acuity testing.

Assessment: Ophthalmoscopy is performed to allow observation of the fundus, i.e., retina, choroid, and sclera and the transparent media, i.e., cornea, aqueous, lens, and vitreous. Changes in color, opacification, and lens position are noted. The retinal vessels, optic disc, and macula are also observed. The presence of myopia or hyperopia can be determined. Hypertension and papilledema can be detected.

Nursing Interventions: Client preparation includes an explanation of the procedure. Clients may be given the opportunity to practice focusing, etc., as part of the examination procedure. The client is informed if mydriatic agents are to be used.

Description of the Procedure: Ophthalmoscopy is performed with inpatients and outpatients. The client may receive a mydriatic medication to dilate the pupils. The client's eyes must be kept open. Client discomfort may arise from the light shining in. Ophthalmoscopic examinations are frequently performed in a darkened room so that lower light levels can be used and discomfort reduced. The examiner may need to use his or her finger to keep the client's eyelids open. The client must fixate on the target. This may be somewhat difficult if the examiner is blocking the target, too much light is present, or the target is very close as in slit-lamp examinations. Both client and examiner must be comfortable to promote the correct angle for observation. The time required for ophthalmoscopy varies. The results are available immediately.

Original Direct Ophthalmoscopy: This technique employs a hand-held ophthalmoscope composed of illuminating, condensing, and focusing systems. An image is placed directly on the client's retina. The examiner is able to visualize a large portion of the client's retina. The examiner's eye is approximately 15 inches from the client.

Indirect (Modern Direct Ophthalmoscopy): This technique uses lenses and a distant light source to examine larger areas of the fundus. The examiner wears a headband light source and places the lens next to the client's eye. The examiner places his or her thumb and little finger on the client's head in order to maintain alignment with the client.

Slit-Lamp Ophthalmoscopy (Biomicroscopy): Slit-lamp ophthalmoscopy is used to examine the small detail of the fundus. A slit lamp is composed of a biomicroscope through which the eye is observed, an illumination system, and a mechanical support system. The client places chin and forehead on the headrest.

Retinoscopy: Retinoscopy produces light and reflects it off a mirror. This allows for examination of the images formed on the retina. The examiner sits back from the client but moves from side to side and forward and backward during the examination.

Keratometer Measurement: The keratometer measures the radius of a portion of the anterior surface of the cornea. This measurement is needed to determine the proper fit for contact lenses and is also used to monitor changes in the shape of the cornea in clients with keratoconus. The client's forehead is supported on the headrest while the examiner uses an eyepiece to see images on the client's retina. A micromatic ophthalmometer is an image doubling device that permits the examination of four images in the client's eye.

Evaluating Client Response: Following the procedure, the client's readiness to deal with ordinary light is assessed. Certain clients may need transportation assistance following administration of some mydriatic agents. Client and family support in dealing with the results is provided.

■ Gonioscopy

Subjective Data: Client complains of poor vision, pain, or inflammation, or may be asymptomatic.

Objective Data: Altered findings on visual acuity testing or ophthalmoscopy.

Assessment: Gonioscopy provides direct visualization of the anterior chamber angle, including the trabecular region where aqueous begins to exit from the eye. Visualization of the chamber angle allows the iris to be seen as it dips down and its base inserts into the ciliary body. The angle is not visualized during ophthalmoscopy. The cornea, pupilary margin, lens, iris, trabecular pigmentation, and Schwalbe's line can also be examined. Gonioscopy is used to differentiae angle closure from open-angle glaucoma and to assess clients with evidence of congenital glaucoma, tumor, or trauma.

Nursing Interventions: Client preparation includes an explanation of the procedure. Client cooperation during lens placement is discussed. Instructions for children can make the procedure seem like a game.

Description of the Procedure: Gonioscopy is performed with inpatients and outpatients. Gonioscopy requires placement of a lens, either a Koeppe lens or a mirrored lens, directly on the eye. Using the Koeppe lens, the client is supine with head turned toward the examiner. As the client looks up, the lower lip of the lens is placed under the lower eyelid. The client then looks down and normal saline or methylcellulose is dripped under the nasal side of the lens to fill the lens–cornea interface.

Using a mirrored lens, the client sits with chin and forehead in the headrest. Solution is placed beneath the client's lower eyelid. The client then looks down and the upper lens lip is placed under the client's upper eyelid. After visualization is completed, the lens is removed. Gonioscopy is completed in less than 15 minutes. The results are available immediately.

Evaluating Client Response: Postprocedure client and family support in dealing with the results is provided.

TONOMETRY

Tonometry provides measurement of intraocular pressure, the hallmark of glaucoma.

Nursing Diagnoses for clients undergoing tonometry include:

- Anxiety related to disease process
- Knowledge deficit related to diagnostic process

Subjective Data: Client complains of loss of peripheral vision or may be asymptomatic.

Objective Data: This is often the first procedure performed.

Assessment: Tonometry is used as a screening tool, particularly for clients over age 40, to diagnose glaucoma and to evaluate response to therapy. Early detection of slight increases in intraocular pressure allow the client to receive appropriate therapy and avoid blindness as a result of untreated glaucoma. Two types of tonometers are in use today. Hand-held impression tonometers measure the depth that a weighted plunger, applied to the cornea, sinks into the eye. Large, mechanical applanation tonometers measure the area of flattening of the cornea when a metal surface is applied. Normal intraocular pressure is 10.5–20.5 mm Hg.

Nursing Interventions: Client preparation includes an explanation of the procedure. Instructions regarding the postanesthetic eye-drop period are discussed.

Description of the Procedure: Tonometry is performed with inpatients and outpatients. The client sits and tilts the head back to receive the anesthetic eye drops. The plunger or weight is applied to the cornea and the pressure reading obtained. Tonometry is completed in less than 5 minutes. The results are available immediately.

Evaluating Client Response: Following the anesthetic eye drops, it is essential the client not scratch or rub the eyes. Children may need extra assistance with this. Client and family support in dealing with the results is provided.

MEASUREMENT OF ELECTRICAL ACTIVITY

- **Electroretinography and Electro-oculography**
- **Electronystagmography**

For clients with impaired sensory input, measurement of electrical activity is used to assess central and peripheral nervous system functioning. A specific consent form may be required.

Nursing Diagnoses for clients undergoing these procedures include:

- Alteration in comfort related to procedure
- Anxiety related to procedure
- Knowledge deficit related to diagnostic process

Electroretinography (ERG) and Electro-oculography (EOG)

Subjective Data: Client complains of problems with vision.

Objective Data: Abnormal vision tests and family history of vision disorders.

Assessment: ERG records electrical activity in the eye in response to light stimuli. It is used for clients with suspected hereditary and constitutional disorders of the retina such as partial and total achromatopsia (color blindness), night blindness, and retinal degeneration such as retinitis pigmentosa, Tay-Sachs Disease, and others. EOG is a recording of these eye movements and is used to complement ERG.

Nursing Interventions: Client education includes an explanation of the procedure. The client is prepared for contact lens and electrode placement.

Description of the Procedure: The procedure is performed with inpatients and outpatients. Children may need extra assistance during this procedure. The client goes to a room specially shielded to eliminate outside electrical interference and other stimuli. For ERG, contact lenses are placed on the client's eyes. Retinal responses to light stimuli are recorded. For EOG, skin electrodes are arranged in pairs around the eyes and taped to the client's face. The client sits in front of a large screen. An array of fluorescent bulbs is behind the screen. Eye movements are first recorded in darkness and then with light adaptation. These procedures take approximately 30 minutes to complete. The results are available following interpretation.

Evaluating Client Response: The client receives eye and skin care following removal of the contact lenses and electrodes. Client and family support in dealing with the results is provided.

■ Electronystagmography (ENG)

Subjective Data: Client complains of syncope and dizziness.

Objective Data: Altered hearing, vision, or neurologic exam.

Assessment: ENG is used to provide objective recordings of vestibular function and thus support diagnostic findings of peripheral or central lesions.

Nursing Interventions: Client education includes an explanation of the procedure. Children may need additional assistance and restraint during this procedure. Electrode placement and the motion involved are discussed. Clients are not allowed seasickness medications such as Dramamine, Marezine, or Bonamine, tranquilizers, caffeine, smoking, or alcohol for 48 hours prior to the test. Anti-convulsant therapy is maintained. Client support for undergoing this procedure is provided. Loosely attached jewelry and prostheses are removed.

Description of the Procedure: ENG is performed on inpatients and outpatients. The ENG battery includes seven tests and is performed in a darkened, quiet room. Initially, the client lies supine. The head may be elevated to 30 degrees. Electrodes are placed at the outer canthus of each eye and extend in a horizontal plane over the pupil. Additional electrodes are placed to run above to below the eye in order to trace vertical nystagmus. A fifth, ground electrode is placed on the scalp. The electrodes are applied with contact paste or gel and are taped to the skin. The battery of ENG tests is performed and requires approximately 1 hour. The results are available following interpretation.

Ocular Dysmetria: The client looks back and forth rapidly.

Fixed Gaze: The client fixates in each of several eye positions for approximately 20 seconds each.

Sinusoidal Tracking Test: The client follows a swinging target.

Optokinetic Nystagmus Test (OKN): The client follows a rotating drum.

Paroxysmal Test: The client's head is moved from a sitting position to a head-lower-than-body position and then to the right. The client is held in this position and recordings obtained for 90 seconds. The client rests for 2–3 minutes in a sitting position and then this maneuver is repeated turning the client's head to the left.

Positional Test: The client is placed in seven different positions, one after another. Recordings are obtained in each position for 60–90 seconds.

Caloric Tests: This procedure is similar to the test discussed in the section, Caloric Stimulation Test but less intensive. Each ear is irrigated in turn for 40 seconds; first with water 7 °C above and then with water 7 °C below body temperature.

Evaluating Client Response: Postprocedure skin care is provided following electrode removal. Fatigue is common and provisions are made for the client to rest. Client and family support in dealing with the procedure and the results is provided.

ULTRASONOGRAPHY

Echography (ultrasonography) is widely used for clinical evaluation of the eye, especially when the media is opaque. No specific consent form is required.

Nursing Diagnoses for clients undergoing echography include:

- Anxiety related to procedure
- Knowledge deficit related to diagnostic process

Subjective Data: Client complains of vision changes, pain, burning, or watering of the eye.

Objective Data: Altered physical exam or visual acuity testing.

Assessment: Echography is used to assess retinal and choroidal detachment, inflammatory or congestive orbital changes, the presence of foreign bodies, intraorbital tumors, and other orbital abnormalities. Ultrasound is also used to obtain accurate biometry of the eye in preparation for prosthetic intraocular lens implants. Two different transducer types are in use: contact real-time scanners that require the use of topical anesthetic eye drops, and immersion systems. In the immersion system, the transducer is suspended in an enclosed water bath that is placed over the client's eye.

Nursing Interventions: The procedure and scanning technique to be used are explained to the client. Specific instructions as to positioning and remaining still during the procedure are provided. If a contact scanner is being used, the client is told not to rub the eyes after the examination since the anesthetized cornea can be damaged.

Description of the Procedure: This procedure is performed with inpatients and outpatients. For echography with a contact real-time scanner, the cornea is anesthetized by means of eye drops. The client sits erect during imaging. For immersion scanning, the client lies supine with the water bath suspended over the eye and surrounding orbit. Echography takes less than 30 minutes to complete. The results are available following interpretation by the ultrasonographer.

Evaluating Client Response: Clients are told not to rub their anesthetized eyes in order to prevent any damage. Children may need extra assistance to prevent rubbing. Client and family support are provided.

RADIOLOGY (LAMINOGRAPHY, TOMOGRAPHY)

For clients with alterations in sensory input, x-rays provide diagnostic data about anatomy and some pathologies. A specific consent form may be required.

Nursing Diagnoses for clients undergoing x-rays include:

- Anxiety related to procedure
- Knowledge deficit related to diagnostic process

Subjective Data: Client complains of recent trauma, hearing loss, tinnitus, and dizziness.

Objective Data: Evidence of recent trauma and altered audiologic or mental status exam.

Assessment: Radiographs detect expansion of the internal auditory canal, which indicates the presence of an acoustic neuroma or other destructive lesion of the temporal bone such as infection, neoplasm, or trauma. Laminography provides more information, but is more costly and exposes the client to higher levels of ionizing radiation. Laminography is used to demonstrate congenital anomalies of the ear and early inflammatory or neoplastic involvement of the temporal bone. It can also reveal trauma to the auditory canal and ossicles and subtle changes associated with otosclerosis and Meniere's disease.

Nursing Interventions: Client education includes an explanation of the procedure. The client wears a hospital gown. All jewelry and prostheses are removed.

Description of the Procedure: This procedure is done with inpatients and outpatients. The client goes to the x-ray department and is positioned according to the view to be obtained. Frequently, more than one radiograph is needed and the client may change position for each view. Clients receive instructions and assistance regarding the desired position and remaining still. Each radiograph is completed in less than 5 minutes. The results are available following interpretation.

Evaluating Client Response: Support for client and family in dealing with the results is provided.

FLUORESCEIN ANGIOGRAPHY

Fluorescein angiography is used to examine the retina. A specific informed consent may be required for this procedure.

Nursing Diagnoses for clients undergoing fluorescein angiography include:

- Alteration in comfort related to procedure
- Anxiety related to procedure
- Knowledge deficit related to diagnostic process

Subjective Data: Client complains of changes in visual fields or pain.

Objective Data: Altered visual acuity testing.

Assessment: Fluorescein angiography is used to detect retinal arterial occlusion, total or partial obstruction, venous turbulence, extravascular blood flow, window defects, retinal pigment epithelial type detachment or diffusing lesions. Sodium fluorescein is administered intravenously. As it passes through the retinal circulation, a fundus camera flash and filter are used to emit light waves in the blue range. This light excites the fluorescein and it responds by emitting green wavelengths that are recorded by the fundus camera.

Nursing Interventions: Client education includes an explanation of the procedure. The client is prepared for the IV injection, the bright lights, and the need to fixate on the target.

Description of the Procedure: This procedure is performed with inpatients and outpatients. Clients go to a darkened room equipped with the fundus camera and flash. A few pictures are taken with the fundus camera to familiarize the client with the bright lights and for practice fixating on the target. Using the antecubital vein, sodium fluorescein 500 mg, in either 5 or 10 ml of solution, is administered as rapidly as possible to obtain a bolus effect. Illumination and photography commence immediately. This procedure is completed in less than 1 hour. Results are available following film processing.

Evaluating Client Response: After the procedure the client is allowed time to readjust to visual stimuli. Client and family support is provided in dealing with the results.

CALORIC STIMULATION TEST (BITHERMAL CALORIC TEST, OCULOVESTIBULAR REFLEX TEST)

This procedure is performed to evaluate vestibular function. A specific consent form may be required.

Nursing Diagnoses for clients undergoing caloric stimulation testing include:

- Alteration in comfort related to procedure
- Anxiety related to procedure
- Knowledge deficit related to diagnostic process

Subjective Data: Client complains of hearing loss, dizziness, and tinnitus.

Objective Data: Altered test results from physical examination and audiologic testing.

Assessment: This procedure is used to assess vestibular functions of the acoustic nerve, to differentiate cerebellar from brainstem function, and to corroborate a suspected diagnosis of Meniere's syndrome or acoustic neuroma. This procedure is contraindicated in clients with perforated tympanic membranes. Normally, clients demonstrate nystagmus and complain of nausea and dizziness within 30 seconds. When cold water is used, nystagmus is downward and away from the irrigated ear. When warm water is inserted, nystagmus is upward toward the irrigated ear.

Nursing Interventions: Client education includes an explanation of the procedure and the expected symptoms, including nausea, vomiting, and dizziness. Clients are told that these symptoms are transitory and will subside after the test and disappear completely in several hours. Clients are NPO 8 hours prior to this procedure to reduce vomiting. Clients are asked to void immediately prior to beginning this procedure. If present during the procedure, the nurse provides emotional support, helps the client maintain a still position, and provides technical assistance as needed.

Description of the Procedure: This procedure is performed with inpatients and outpatients. Determination is made that the client's eardrums are intact. The client either sits with the head tilted forward at a 30 degree angle or is horizontal with the head tilted backward at a 60 degree angle. The client assumes a fixed stare and is draped. The affected side is tested first. Cold fluid, 7 °C or more below body temperature, is directed into the auditory canal. This procedure is repeated as both ears are tested with fluid of different temperatures. The auditory canal is irrigated with 250 ml of fluid for 30 seconds, until symptoms appear, or for a maximum of 3 minutes. There is a 5-minute wait between each ear irrigation. After the test is finished, the client is dried and the drapes are removed. This procedure takes less than 30 minutes to complete. The results are available immediately.

Evaluating Client Response: Following the procedure, the client is maintained on bed rest for 1–3 hours. Food and medication are resumed. The client is observed for nausea, vomiting, or dizziness. Safety measures, such as raising side rails, are implemented. The room is kept quiet and nonstimulating. Usual activities of daily living are resumed when symptoms have disappeared. Client and family support in dealing with the results is provided.

9

Clients with Sexual Dysfunction

Clients with sexual dysfunction undergoing the diagnostic process need much nursing support, not only because of pathophysiology, but also because of society's reactions to sexuality and sexual problems. Client knowledge in this area may be skewed. The diagnostic process itself can threaten the self-esteem of clients. Nursing diagnoses for clients during the diagnostic process focus on psychosocial needs as well as pathophysiologic concerns.

For clients with sexual dysfunction, significant data is revealed by physical examination. A thorough personal history and history of the present illness are mandatory. A detailed recording of the client's subjective comments is obtained. The examiner must be comfortable in asking questions and hearing the responses. Clients sense the examiner's professionalism and are more apt to answer what is asked. Physical examination should not be considered complete unless the client has been taught monthly self-examination of the breasts or testes.

Breast self-examination (BSE) is best performed a few days after completion of menstruation, when the breasts have less fluid and are less tender. BSE begins with inspecting the breasts in the mirror. Normal breasts are symmetrical, however some variation in size is common. The breasts are observed for redness, dimpling, flattening, or lumps. Long-standing inversion of the nipples is common and normal. Discharge or change in nipple shape is not normal and is noted. The client should raise and lower her arms and again inspect her breasts for symmetry, retraction or dimpling. Palpation should be performed with the client both sitting and lying down. The client places her left arm behind her head while examining the left breast and vice versa. Each breast is palpated in a systematic, circular manner using three fingers to compress the tissue against the chest wall. The nipples are compressed between thumb and forefinger and observed for discharge. The axilla are also palpated. Clients are taught to contact a health professional if any changes or unusual findings are noted.

The Papanicolaou (Pap) Smear is conducted on a routine annual basis. This test consists of three specimens. No lubricant other than water is used on the speculum. Smears are obtained before palpation to avoid distortion of the findings.

The endocervical smear is obtained by using a cotton swab moistened with saline. The swab is rolled clockwise and counterclockwise on the cervical os. It is removed and gently wiped onto a glass slide. The slide is fixed at once.

The cervical scrape uses a scraping of the cervical os. The scraper is then gently wiped onto a glass slide and fixed.

The vaginal pool is wiped with a dry cotton swab that is then rolled gently on a glass slide and fixed.

Testicular self-examination should be performed on a regular basis. The penis, prepuce or foreskin, glans, and urethral meatus are inspected for color, ulceration, nodule, or discharge. The scrotum and its contour are also inspected. Each testis and epididymis is palpated for size, shape, and consistency. Each spermatic cord and vas deferens is palpated for nodules or swelling. Clients are taught to contact a health professional if any changes or unusual findings are noted.

LABORATORY TESTS

The underlying pathophysiology of sexual dysfunction may be assessed through laboratory tests. Client cooperation enhances the efficient use of time, resources, and cost during the diagnostic process.

Nursing Diagnoses for clients undergoing laboratory tests include:

- Anxiety related to procedure
- Knowledge deficit related to diagnostic process

LABORATORY TESTS

Test	Purpose	Normal Values	Nursing Actions
Acid phosphatase	Assess		
Serum	prostate status, Paget's disease, multiple myeloma, parathyroid or renal function	Adult: <4.0 ng/ml	
Vaginal aspirate	Assessment in alleged rape		High level in seminal fluid
Androstanedione Serum	Assess hirsutism, ovary function	0.6–3 μg/ml in premenopausal women	Specimen is collected 1 wk before or after menstruation
Alphafetoprotein (AFP) Serum	Assess hepatic, testicular, carcinoma	0–10 ng/ml	
	Assess fetus for open neural tube defects	Considered elevated at 2.5 times the median AFP value	At least two samples with elevated levels

(Continued)

LABORATORY TESTS (cont.)

Test	Purpose	Normal Values	Nursing Actions
AFP (cont.)		for each gestational wk	are needed for diagnostic accuracy
Estrogens Serum and urine	Assess ovarian function, pregnancy and fetal distress	Ovulation: 28–100 μg Luteal phase: 22–105 μg Menses: 4–25 μg Pregnancy: up to 45,000 μg Post menopause: 14–20 μg	Done serially to determine gradual rise during pregnancy Accurate menstrual history needed for analysis of results
Estrone (E1)		Serum: 2–25 μg Urine: 2–25 mg/24 hrs	Collection container is kept in the refrigerator
Estradiol (E2)		Serum: 1–10 μg Urine: 0–10 mg/24 hrs	
Estriol (E3)		Serum: 2–30 μg Urine: 1–25 mg	Value is related to wk of gestation
Follicle stimulating hormone (FSH) Serum	Assess level, anterior pituitary function	Female: nonovulating: 5–18 mU/ml oral contraceptives: 0–10 mU/ml pregnant: 0–3 mU/ml postmenopausal: 30–300 mU/ml Male: 5–18 mU/ml	
Urine		Female: related to menstrual phase: 5–100 IU/24 hr	Container must contain preservative or be

LABORATORY TESTS (cont.)

Test	Purpose	Normal Values	Nursing Actions
FSH (cont.)		Male: 5–25 IU/24 hr	kept on ice
Gonorrhea culture Vagina Urethra Anus Throat	Determine presence of pathogen	Negative	
Human chorionic gonadotropin (HCG) Serum	Assess testicular carcinoma	None present	
17 Ketosteroids Urine	Assess adrenal, testicular function	Adult female: 5–15 mg/24 hr Adult male: 8–20 mg/24 hr Child: <3 mg/24 hr Infant: <1 mg/24 hr	Preservative in container and ice on the outside are required
Luteinizing hormone (LH) Serum	Assess level, pituitary function	Female: nonovulating: 5–30 mU/ml oral contraceptives: 2–12 mU/ml postmenopausal: 25–150 mU/ml Male: 4–20 mU/ml	
Urine		Female: related to menstrual phase: 2–110 IU/24 hr Male: 5–18 IU/24 hr	Collection container must contain preservative or be kept on ice
Pregnancy test (placental hormone test, HCG) Serum or blood	Assess presence of hormone, indicating pregnancy	Negative	

(Continued)

LABORATORY TESTS (cont.)

Test	Purpose	Normal Values	Nursing Actions
Pregnanediol Urine	Assess progesterone level, fertility, Addison's disease	Proliferation: 0.5–1.5 mg/24 hr Luteal: 2–7 mg/24 hr Postmenopausal: 0.2–1.0 mg/24 hr	Collection container must contain preservative or be kept on ice
Prostatic acid phosphate (PAP) Serum	Assess prostate, tumor marker	1.399–9.839 ng/ml	
Syphilis detection (FTA-ABS, flourescent antibody, TP-MHA, hemagglutination, RPR, VDRL, complement fixation flocculation) Serum	Identify organism	Negative, nonreactive	
Testosterone	Determine level	Female: prepuberty: 10–20 ng/100 ml menstrual: 20–80 ng/100 ml postmenopausal: 8–35 ng/100 ml Male: prepuberty: 10–20 ng/100 ml adult: 300–1000 ng/100 ml	

Please note, these values are guidelines. Check with the laboratory performing the test for absolute values.

ULTRASONOGRAPHY

Ultrasound is a major diagnostic tool for clients with sexual dysfunction because it does not involve ionizing radiation. Dedicated, or use-specific ultrasonography permits sensitive and accurate interpretation. No specific consent form is required.

Nursing Diagnoses for clients undergoing ultrasound include:

- Alteration in comfort, bladder distension related to procedure
- Anxiety related to procedure
- Knowledge deficit related to diagnostic process

Subjective Data: Nonpregnant female clients may complain of bleeding, pain, or fertility difficulties. Male clients may complain of tenderness.

Objective Data: Pregnancy, history of trauma, or altered physical findings in breast tissue, pelvic area, or testicles.

Assessment: Ultrasound mammography is used for women who present with a palpable mass, dense glandular tissue as demonstrated on x-ray, clinically equivocal physical findings, inflammatory breast disease, breast augmentation, or pregnancy. Dedicated real-time ultrasound equipment is of two types. Water bath scanners require the client to be prone with breasts suspended in the water bath. Scanning is done through the water to prevent the glandular tissue from moving. High-resolution contact scanners are also used, especially for younger women with dense breasts. For this type of scanner, the breast is compressed against the chest wall to allow determination of solid and cystic masses.

Pelvic ultrasound is used with clients with clinical evidence of pelvic mass, pelvic inflammatory disease, endometriosis, gynecologic malignancy, or misplaced intrauterine device.

Obstetrical ultrasound is a widely used diagnostic procedure. It is used to diagnose pregnancy, determine gestational age, diagnose multiple pregnancies, assess vaginal bleeding during pregnancy, diagnose hydatidiform mole, diagnose extrauterine pregnancy, locate and assess anomalies of the placenta, assess fetal growth, diagnose fetal anomalies, determine fetal death, aid in amniocentesis, and assess induced abortion and postpartum complications. A full bladder is a prerequisite for pelvic sonograms. The bladder acts as a window to the uterus and displaces it away from the bowel. Various ultrasonic techniques are used, such as gray-scale and real-time, depending on individual requirements. Doppler ultrasound, which requires no client preparation, is available in some obstetrical offices.

Ultrasound is used to assess male clients with scrotal swelling or masses. Intratesticular lesions are differentiated from extratesticular lesions. Ultrasonography can identify intratesticular hemorrhage, hydroceles, and whether the testicle is intact after trauma. In newborn or pediatric clients, ultrasound is used to determine testicular descent. This procedure requires water bath scanning.

Nursing Interventions: Client education includes specific instruction as to the type of scanner used, positioning, remaining still, and feeling some pressure during the procedure. For pelvic examinations, the nurse provides the client with instruction regarding a full bladder and access to a bathroom following the procedure. Clients are prepared for potential difficulty in not urinating during the procedure.

Description of the Procedure: Ultrasound is performed with inpatients and outpatients. Privacy is assured. The client assumes the required position. For contact scanners, conductive oil or gel is applied for optimal contact between transducer and skin. The transducer is moved across the skin area according to the type of sonogram being performed. Ultrasound examinations take approximately 30 minutes to complete. The results are available following interpretation.

Evaluating Client Response: The results of sonograms may be given to the client at the time of examination. Client and family support in dealing with the results is provided.

MAGNETIC RESONANCE IMAGING (MR, Nuclear Magnetic Imaging, NMR)

The use of MR for clients with sexual dysfunction is being refined. MR is preferred to CT since MR does not involve ionizing radiation or contrast medium. A specific consent form may be required.

Nursing Diagnoses for clients undergoing MR include:

- Anxiety related to procedure
- Knowledge deficit related to diagnostic process

Subjective Data: Client complains of pain or unusual bleeding.

Objective Data: Altered physical exam or laboratory data.

Assessment: Use of MR in examining the breasts is thus far limited. In the pelvis, MR is used to delineate myometrium and endometrium. The vagina can be visualized separately from the uterus, rectum, and bladder. The normal prostate visualizes well, particularly in relation to the bladder. MR is contraindicated in clients with aneurysm clips anywhere in the body or with pacemakers because of the effects of the magnetic field.

Nursing Interventions: Client education includes the need to remain still during imaging. Clients are prepared for the imposing size of the MR scanner and the noninvasive nature of the procedure is emphasized. A client health history specific to past insertion of aneurysm clips or pacemaker is obtained. The client changes into a hospital gown, removes all jewelry and prostheses, and voids prior to the procedure.

Description of the Procedure: MR is performed with inpatients and outpatients. The client goes to the MR room. The client is supine within the body scanner during the scanning procedure. Completion time depends upon image quality and may take up to 1 hour. Results are available after interpretation.

Evaluating Client Response: Postprocedure client and family support in dealing with the results is provided.

RADIOLOGY

Mammography is widely used as a screening tool and for individual diagnosis. A specific consent form may be required.

Nursing Diagnoses for the client undergoing mammography include:

- Anxiety related to procedure
- Knowledge deficit related to diagnostic process

Subjective Data: Client complains of pain, tenderness, or a lump.

Objective Data: Altered physical data, including palpation of a mass or change in breast size, shape, or skin configuration.

Assessment: Mammography is the "gold standard" for the diagnosis of breast cancer. Mammography demonstrates minimal breast cancer, i.e., carcinoma in situ or invasive carcinoma of less than 5 mm. It also detects microcalcifications that herald developing breast cancer. Xeromammography is a mammographic technique that provides superior imaging of microcalcifications, but requires a higher dose of radiation. Statistics indicate a 5-year survival rate of 93% for women with nonpalpable cancers found by mammographic screening. Concern over ionizing radiation exposure has been voiced since the 1960s. However, current "dedicated" equipment uses significantly lower radiation doses than were used previously. Mammography is also used to determine the presence of benign breast disease, cysts, fibroadenomas, cystosarcomas, medullary carcinomas, and to guide needle biopsy. Thermography, photography using heat sensitive film, may be used as adjunct procedure following mammography, especially for clients with dense breasts. Thermography does not replace mammography. Clients undergoing mammography may have detected a lump themselves, had a mass detected on routine physical examination, or may be undergoing screening.

X-ray pelvimetry may be performed late in pregnancy if clinical pelvimetry is equivocal, when abnormal presentation and position are evidenced, when labor is prolonged, or if abnormal development of the fetus is suspected. X-ray pelvimetry is performed less frequently, as ultrasound is more widely used.

Nursing Interventions: Nursing actions prior to the procedure include an explanation of the procedure. For mammography, caffeine intake may be limited 2 weeks prior to the procedure. Client education includes providing lists of the many sources of caffeine, e.g., coffee, tea, cola, cocoa, medications, etc. All jewelry, prostheses, etc., are removed. During x-ray pelvimetry, the client is accompanied by an obstetrical nurse for reassurance and assistance in positioning. Emergency obstetrical equipment is available.

For the purpose of client education, the indications for mammography as issued in 1984 by The American Cancer Society and the American College of Radiology are listed. They state that mammography is indicated for:

1. All clients with any sign or symptom suggestive of breast carcinoma;
2. All women over the age of 50 annually, regardless of the presence or absence of symptoms;
3. All women by age 40 as a baseline; and
4. Women in high-risk categories after consultation with a physician to discuss obtaining baseline or annual mammograms at an earlier age.

   The American College of Radiology further recommends mammographic screening of asymptomatic women between ages 40 and 50 at 1–2 year intervals.

Description of the Procedure: Mammography is performed with inpatients and outpatients. Privacy is assured. Mammograms are obtained in different positions. The client is placed between the camera and the film as each breast is compressed for a clearer image. Mammography is completed in approximately 30 minutes. X-ray pelvimetry is performed with the client supine on the examining table and takes less than 10 minutes. The results are available following interpretation.

Evaluating Client Response: Postprocedure support for client and family in dealing with the results is provided.

COMPUTED TOMOGRAPHY (CT, COMPUTERIZED AXIAL TOMOGRAPHY, CAT SCAN, EMI)

CT has limited use for clients with sexual dysfunction. A specific consent form may be required.

Nursing Diagnoses for clients undergoing CT include:

- Anxiety related to procedure
- Knowledge deficit related to diagnostic process
- Potential for injury: allergic reaction related to procedure

Subjective Data: Client complains of changes in breast tissue.

Objective Data: Clinical evidence highly suggestive of breast cancer, such as the presence of a breast lump or other prior test results suggestive of breast disease.

Assessment: CT has some use in clients with suspected breast cancer. The higher levels of ionizing radiation and the need for contrast medium make this technique an inappropriate screening device. However, diseased breast tissue contains higher levels of iodine and iodide than does normal breast tissue and shows a marked degree of enhancement following iodinated contrast medium administration. Thus, CT is used for women with radiographically dense breasts, in whom a lesion is not clearly seen, or in whom a suspected primary lesion cannot be localized.

Nursing Interventions: Client education prior to CT scanning includes an explanation of the procedure and the need to remain still during imaging. The imposing size of the CT scanner is explained and the noninvasive nature of the procedure is emphasized. If the client is undergoing a contrast-enhanced scan, a history specific as to allergy to iodine or previous reaction to contrast medium is elicited. Clients are frequently NPO 2–4 hours prior to contrast-enhanced CT scans. Clear liquids may be permitted. The client changes into a hospital gown, removes all jewelry and prostheses.

Description of the Procedure: CT is performed with inpatients and outpatients. The client goes to the CT room. IV administration of contrast medium may precede CT scanning by 1 hour. The client is supine on the gantry during the scanning procedure. Suspended respiration is not required. Scanning time is less than 20 minutes. Results are available after interpretation.

Evaluating Client Response: Fluid intake is encouraged to assist in eliminating the contrast medium. Medication administration is resumed. Postprocedure client and family support in dealing with the results is provided.

DIRECT VISUALIZATION

- Colposcopy
- Hysteroscopy
- Culdoscopy
- Laparoscopy

For clients with sexual dysfunction, several different direct visualization techniques are in use. A specific consent form may be required for these procedures.

Nursing Diagnoses for clients undergoing direct visualization include:

- Alteration in comfort related to procedure
- Anxiety related to procedure
- Knowledge deficit related to diagnostic process
- Potential loss of pregnancy related to procedure

Colposcopy (Colpomicroscopy, Cervical Biopsy)

Subjective Data: Client complains of pain, tenderness, or unusual bleeding.

Objective Data: Altered physical exam, Pap smear, history of hormone use by the client's mother, and abnormal laboratory findings.

Assessment: Colposcopy provides direct examination of the vagina, vulva, and cervical epithelium. This procedure may follow a suspicious Pap smear and is done to obtain a cervical punch biopsy, assess dysplasia, leukoplakia, abnormal blood vessels, or to stage carcinoma. Colposcopy is considered safe for use with pregnant women. Colposcopy may also be used for biopsy excision of an inverted cone of tissue. If so, IV sedation is usually required and the procedure is performed in an operating room.

Nursing Interactions: Client education includes an explanation of the procedure and the need to remain still. If this procedure is to be performed in the operating room, appropriate presurgical and anesthesia nursing responsibilities are implemented. If present during colposcopy, the nurse provides client reassurance and technical assistance.

Description of the Procedure: This procedure is performed with inpatients and outpatients. Privacy is assured. Colposcopy is performed with the client in the lithotomy position. The colposcope is inserted into the vagina and advanced toward the cervix. The light source permits detailed visual inspection of the mucosa. The client may experience some pressure or pain when the biopsy specimen is obtained. The colposcope is withdrawn and the procedure completed in less than 20 minutes. Visualization results are available immediately; biopsy results are available following interpretation.

Evaluating Client Response: Vital signs are monitored. Packing may be placed following biopsy and is left in place for 8–24 hours. If this procedure was performed in the operating room, appropriate postsurgical and anesthesia nursing responsibilities are implemented. The client is instructed not to engage in sexual intercourse for several days and to report excessive bleeding to the physician. Client and family support in dealing with the results is provided.

■ Hysteroscopy

Subjective Data: Client complains of infertility, pain, tenderness, or unusual bleeding.

Objective Data: Altered physical exam.

Assessment: Hysteroscopy permits direct visualization of the uterine cavity. It is most commonly used to assess clients with infertility, unexplained bleeding, or retained IUD. Hysteroscopy is best performed on day 5 of the menstrual cycle. Hysteroscopy is contraindicated in clients with cervical or endometrial carcinoma.

Nursing Interventions: Client education includes an explanation of the procedure and the need to remain still. If present during hysteroscopy, the nurse provides client reassurance and technical assistance.

Description of the Procedure: Hysteroscopy is performed with inpatients and outpatients. Privacy is provided. Hysteroscopy is performed with the client in the lithotomy position. The vagina and vulva are prepared and a paracervical anesthetic block is administered. The hysteroscope is passed through the vagina and advanced 1–2 cm into the cervical canal. Sterile solution is inserted through the hysteroscope to dilate the uterus and allow for complete inspection. After visualization is complete, the fluid is drained and the hysteroscope removed. This procedure is completed in 30–60 minutes. Visualization results are available immediately.

Evaluating Client Response: Postprocedure client and family support in dealing with the results is provided. Rest is provided for the client as the anesthetic effects subside.

■ Culdoscopy

Subjective Data: Client complains of infertility, pain, tenderness, or unusual bleeding.

Objective Data: Altered physical findings.

Assessment: Culdoscopy permits observation of the uterus, fallopian tubes, ovaries, broad ligaments, rectal wall, and sigmoid colon from inside the cul-de-sac. It is used for client with suspected infertility from fallopian tube abnormality or to visualize an ectopic pregnancy or pelvic mass. Culdoscopy is contraindicated in clients with acute vaginal or vulvular infection, peritonitis, or adhesions of bowel to cul-de-sac from prior surgery.

Nursing Interventions: Client education includes an explanation of the procedure and positioning. If this procedure is to be performed in the operating room, appropriate presurgical and anesthesia nursing responsibilities are implemented. If present during culdoscopy, the nurse provides client reassurance and technical assistance.

Description of the Procedure: Culdoscopy is performed with inpatients and outpatients. Local, regional, or general anesthesia may be used. The client is placed in a knee-to-chest position. A surgical incision is made in the posterior vagina wall. The culdoscope is inserted into the vagina and passed through the incision into the cul-de-sac. It is rotated to provide the desired visualization and withdrawn when the examination is complete. Sutures are not needed for incisional healing. Culdoscopy is complete in approximately 1 hour. Visualization results are available immediately.

Evaluating Client Response: Vital signs are monitored. If this procedure was performed under general anesthesia, appropriate postsurgical nursing responsibilities are implemented. The client is assessed for excessive bleeding and told to report any future excessive bleeding to the physician. The client is instructed not to engage in sexual intercourse or douching for 2 weeks. Client and family support in dealing with the results is provided.

■ Laparoscopy (Pelvic Endoscopy, Pelvic Peritoneoscopy)

Subjective Data: Client complains of pain, cramping, tenderness, or unusual bleeding.

Objective Data: Altered findings on physical exam from laboratory and other diagnostic tests.

Assessment: Laparoscopy is performed on clients with clinical evidence of adhesions, endometriosis, cysts, or masses in order to visualize the pelvis and intestines. Clients may present with symptoms of gastrointestinal or reproductive disorders. An ovarian biopsy or other minor surgical procedures, such as tubal ligation or lysis of adhesions, may be performed as part of laparoscopy.

Nursing Interventions: Preprocedure nursing responsibilities include an explanation of the procedure and positioning. If this procedure is to be performed under general anesthesia, appropriate presurgical nursing responsibilities are implemented. All jewelry and prostheses are removed.

Description of the Procedure: Laparoscopy is performed with inpatients and outpatients. The client is placed supine on the operating room table and receives IV sedation or general anesthesia. The anterior abdominal wall entry site, commonly near the left iliac fossa or in the midline below the umbilicus, is located and prepared. Local anesthesia is administered as needed. A surgical incision is made and a trocar is inserted and then aspirated to ensure that intestine or large vessels have not been perforated. Nitrous oxide or carbon dioxide may be inserted to create a pneumoperitoneum. This permits better visualization by separating the pelvic organs from the intestines. A uterine cannula may be inserted into the uterus to position it for better visualization. The laparoscope may be inserted through the first incision or through a second incision. After visualization is complete, the laparoscope is removed. The trocar is removed after the air has diffused from the peritoneum. The incision is sutured closed and a dressing applied. Laparoscopy requires approximately 1 hour. Visualization results are available immediately.

Evaluating Client Response: Vital signs are monitored. If laparoscopy was performed under general anesthesia, appropriate nursing responsibilities are implemented. Abdominal discomfort resulting from gaseous distension and organ manipulation is common and is to be expected. Pain medications are administered as needed. Severe, more persistent pain may be indicative of bleeding within the peritoneal ligaments or mesentery, or at the biopsy site and is reported to the physician. Client and family support in dealing with the results is provided.

BIOPSY

- **Breast Biopsy**
- **Endometrial Smear**

Biopsy is the definitive diagnostic method for many pathophysiologies. A specific consent form is required for these procedures.

Nursing Diagnoses for clients undergoing biopsy include:

- Alteration in comfort related to procedure
- Anxiety related to procedure
- Knowledge deficit related to diagnostic process

Breast Biopsy (Needle Biopsy)

Subjective Data: Client complains of pain, tenderness, or discharge.

Objective Data: Altered physical exam or abnormal results from mammography.

Assessment: The presence of a palpable lump is the primary indication for breast biopsy.

Nursing Interventions: Client education includes an explanation of the procedure. Client support during the diagnostic process is provided.

Description of the Procedure: Breast needle biopsy is performed with inpatients and outpatients. Privacy is provided. Ultrasonography or mammography may be used to guide needle insertion. Local anesthetic may be administered intradermally and subcutaneously at the entry site. The needle is inserted and then suction may be used to aspirate tissue into the syringe. The needle is withdrawn. The procedure is completed in less than 10 minutes. The results are available following interpretation.

Evaluating Client Response: Following the procedure, the client is monitored for bleeding at the entry site. Analgesics are administered as needed. Client and family support in dealing with the results is provided.

Endometrial Smear (Endometrial Aspiration, Endometrial Biopsy)

Subjective Data: Client complains of pain, tenderness, or unusual bleeding.

Objective Data: Altered physical exam and abnormal results from other tests.

Assessment: Endometrial smear or aspiration is used to screen clients at risk for carcinoma. Endometrial biopsy provides definitive histoctyologic diagnosis and staging.

Nursing Interventions: Client education includes an explanation of the procedure. Client support for the diagnostic process is provided.

Description of the Procedure: These procedures are performed with inpatients and outpatients. Privacy is provided. The client assumes the lithotomy position on the examining table. For an endometrial smear, a cannula is inserted into the endometrial cavity. The cannula is connected to a syringe attached to a collecting receptical. Isotonic saline is inserted. Then, mild negative pressure is created so that tissue and fluid can be aspirated. Endometrial aspiration involves the use of a suction curettage with the distal tip inserted into the uterine cavity. Negative pressure is created and tissue is aspirated into a collection container at the proximal end of the curettage. For endometrial biopsy, intrauterine local anesthetic is administered and a curette used to biopsy the tissue. Suction may be used to obtain the tissue sample. These procedures are completed in less than 15 minutes. The results are available following interpretation.

Evaluating Client Response: Following the procedure, the client is monitored for bleeding. Profuse bleeding or severe pain are reported to the physician. Analgesics are administered as needed. Client and family support in dealing with the results is provided.

10

Clients with Potential Alteration in Family Process

Most parents look joyfully toward pregnancy and healthy babies. For many parents, however, pregnancy comes either with difficulty or with potentially serious complications for child and family.

Infertility affects many couples. Determination of the contributing factors includes laboratory studies in addition to the tests in this section. Meeting the emotional needs of these clients is a major nursing goal. The clients' self-concepts may be severely affected by infertility, and the procedures require changes in usually private activities.

The birth process is a major event, psychologically and physiologically. Testing is available today that is used as one predictive factor in determining the need for and type of interventions that may be employed to enhance the birth process.

Infants with congenital defects or birth anomalies have a major impact on their families. Many families with related past personal or family histories choose to test the fetuses before birth. There are major implications of the results for the child, the parents, and family.

FERTILITY TESTS

- **Seminal Fluid Analysis**
- **Testicular Scan**
- **Sims-Huhner Test**
- **Rubin's Test**

For clients who have been unable to conceive, these tests are the first steps of a fertility workup. A specific consent form may be required.

Nursing Diagnoses for clients undergoing fertility tests include:

- Alteration in family dynamics related to procedure
- Alteration in comfort related to procedure
- Anxiety related to procedure
- Knowledge deficit related to diagnostic process

Seminal Fluid Analysis (Semen Test, Sperm Count)

Subjective Data: Clients present with a history of infertility.

Objective Data: Presence of infertility.

Assessment: In order to examine the "seminal factor" in infertility, analysis is made of the ejaculate. Sperm counts are done to determine the effectiveness of a vasectomy.

Normal Values:

Volume: 2–5 ml.
Count: 60–200 million.
Motility: 70–80% active.
Morphology: 60–80% correct shape.

Nursing Interventions: Client education emphasizes the importance of time intervals for specimen collection and examination. The client is told to keep the specimen at room temperature during transport. Containers may be provided.

Description of the Procedure: This procedure is performed with outpatients. This test is scheduled in advance. At least 3 days should elapse between the client's last ejaculation and the ejaculation used for analysis.

The client ejaculates into a clean dry container. The sample must be kept at room temperature and is examined microscopically within 2–4 hours.

Evaluating Client Response: Postprocedure support for client and family is provided.

■ Testicular Scan

Subjective Data: Clients present with a history of infertility.

Objective Data: Presence of infertility.

Assessment: This scintigraphic study is used to determine if varices within the testicles are a contributing factor in infertility. It may also be used in clients with suspected testicular carcinoma.

Nursing Interventions: Client education includes an explanation of the procedure and the required positioning. Scheduling considerations include 24–48 hours between different scintigraphic procedures to reduce potential cross-interference.

Description of the Procedure: This procedure is performed with inpatients and outpatients. The client's penis is taped to the abdomen and the testicles are placed under the scintillation camera to permit accurate imaging. The radiopharmaceutical is injected intravenously and imaging begins. This procedure is completed in 1 hour. The results are available following interpretation.

Evaluating Client Response: Postprocedure support for client and family is provided.

■ Sims-Huhner Test (P-K Test)

Subjective Data: Clients present with a history of infertility.

Objective Data: Altered physical exam including basal temperature chart.

Assessment: This test is done to assess the "cervical factor" in infertility. It is performed 1–2 hours after the couple has had intercourse and may be scheduled to coincide with ovulation.

Nursing Interventions: Client education includes an explanation of the procedure and the importance of time between intercourse and the office visit. Restrictions during this period, i.e., the woman not voiding, bathing, or douching are discussed. If present during the procedure, the nurse provides emotional support, helps the client maintain a still position, and provides technical assistance.

Description of the Procedure: This procedure is performed with outpatients and is scheduled in advance. The couple has intercourse. The woman may be asked to remain on her back with hips elevated for approximately 30 minutes. The woman must arrive at the physician's office within 1–2 hours after intercourse. During this time period, she wears a perineal pad and does not void, bathe, or douche. Clients are assured privacy and assume the lithotomy position on the examining table. Using a small dropper, cervical contents are aspirated. These secretions are examined under a microscope for presence and viability of sperm. The results are available immediately.

Evaluating Client Response: Following the procedure, the client gets dressed. Client and spouse support is provided as needed.

■ Rubin's Test (Tubal Insufflation)

Subjective Data: Clients present with a history of infertility.

Objective Data: Altered physical exam including basal temperature chart.

Assessment: This test is done to determine the "tubal factor" in infertility. With the use of carbon dioxide, tubal patency is determined. If the pressure gauge reaches 200 mm Hg, the tubes are considered occluded.

Nursing Interventions: Client education includes an explanation of the procedure. Clients are prepared for potential discomfort during and after the procedure. The use of analgesia is discussed. If present during the procedure, the nurse provides emotional support, helps the client maintain a still position, and provides technical assistance.

Description of the Procedure: This test is performed with inpatients and outpatients. Privacy is provided. The client assumes the lithotomy position on the examining table. The client may receive atropine to reduce tubal spasm. A sterile cannula is inserted in the vagina and passed into the uterus. Carbon dioxide is inserted into the uterus. As the air travels up the fallopian tubes and into the peritoneal cavity, the physician listens to the abdomen with a stethoscope. If the fallopian tubes are patent, the physician will hear gas in the abdomen. The client may experience referred pain under the scapula or shoulder on the same side as the open tube. The procedure is completed in approximately 1 hour. The results are available immediately.

Evaluating Client Response: Following the procedure, the client rests for several hours. Complaints of cramping, shoulder pain, dizziness, and nausea are common. The client may find that lying on her abdomen with pelvis higher than her head will reduce discomfort by allowing the gas to rise in the pelvis. Analgesics are administered as needed. Emotional support is provided for client and spouse.

CONTRAST STUDIES

- **Hysterosalpingogram**
- **Vesiculogram**

For clients with infertility, contrast studies are a means of examining pelvic structures. A specific consent form is required for these procedures.

Nursing Diagnoses for clients undergoing contrast studies include:

- Alteration in comfort related to procedure
- Anxiety related to procedure
- Knowledge deficit related to diagnostic process
- Potential for injury: allergic reaction related to procedure

Hysterosalpingogram (Uterotubogram)

Subjective Data: Clients present with a history of infertility.

Objective Data: Altered data from physical exam and other diagnostic tests.

Assessment: This procedure evaluates tubal patency and the presence of uterine pathology in clients with a history of infertility or repeated spontaneous abortion. The contrast medium is a water-soluble iodine-based solution. It is contraindicated for clients who are pregnant or who have an active pelvic infection.

Nursing Interventions: Client education includes explanation of the procedure and the client's role. The client is prepared for some discomfort. A client history specific for pregnancy, allergy to iodine, and previous reaction to contrast medium is obtained. Prior to the procedure, clients may receive bowel preparation, cathartics, and/or enemas to eliminate gas shadows from the radiographs. Analgesics may be given to prevent and/or reduce discomfort during the procedure. The client wears a hospital gown, removes all jewelry and prostheses.

Description of the Procedure: This procedure is performed with inpatients and outpatients. The client assumes the lithotomy position on the radiology table. A bivalved speculum is inserted into the vagina and advanced to reveal the cervix. A cannula is inserted into the uterine cavity and/or fallopian tubes and radiopaque contrast medium is inserted. Serial radiographs are obtained. A Hysterosalpingogram is completed in approximately 1 hour. Preliminary results may be available immediately, but definitive diagnosis may require extensive viewing of the films.

Evaluating Client Response: Vital signs are monitored. Analgesics are provided as needed. Clients are encouraged to wear a sanitary pad for several hours since the contrast medium may stain clothing. Client and family support in dealing with the results and the need for any further testing is provided.

■ Vesiculogram

Subjective Data: Clients present with a history of infertility.

Objective Data: Altered data from physical exam and other diagnostic tests.

Assessment: Vesiculography is performed to evaluate infertility. It requires surgical exposure of the vas deferens and the use of a contrast medium containing iodine.

Nursing Interventions: Client education includes an explanation of the procedure. The effects of local anesthesia are discussed. The client is prepared for some discomfort. A client history specific to allergy to iodine or previous reaction to contrast medium is obtained. Clients remove all jewelry and prostheses and wear a hospital gown.

Description of the Procedure: This procedure is performed with inpatients and outpatients. The client goes to the radiology department and lies supine on the radiology table. The incision site is located and prepared. Local anesthetic is administered and a small incision is made into the vas deferens. Contrast medium is inserted into the vas and the seminal vesicles. Serial radiographs are obtained. Vesiculography is completed in approximately 1 hour. Preliminary results may be available immediately, but definitive diagnosis may require repeated viewing of the films.

Evaluating Client Response: The incision site is monitored for bleeding. Analgesics are provided as needed. The client is told that contrast medium may stain clothing. Client and family support in dealing with the results is provided.

FETAL TESTING

- **Nonstress Testing**
- **Oxytocin Challenge Test**

When it is suspected that a fetus is at risk, fetal testing is used to obtain more data. These procedures are performed on mothers who are at risk for placental insufficiency or difficulty during labor. A specific consent form may be required.

Nursing Diagnoses for clients undergoing fetal testing include:

- Alteration in comfort related to procedure
- Anxiety related to procedure
- Knowledge deficit related to diagnostic process
- Potential for pregnancy complications related to procedure

Nonstress Testing (NST, Fetal Acceleration Determination)

Objective Data: Abnormal fetal findings or abnormal or difficult to analyze maternal laboratory findings, particularly estriol levels.

Assessment: Nonstress testing records the fetal heart rate. The recording is analyzed in terms of fetal activity, acceleration of the fetal heart rate during fetal activity, baseline variability of the fetal heart rate and uterine activity.

Nursing Interventions: Client education includes an explanation of the procedure. If present during the procedure, the nurse provides emotional support, helps the client maintain a still position, and provides technical assistance.

Description of the Procedure: NST is performed with inpatients and outpatients. Privacy is provided. An ultrasonic or phototransducer is placed on the mother's abdomen to record the fetal heart rate and a pressure transducer is placed over the area of the fundus to record uterine contractions. The client is monitored for 30–40 minutes. The results are available immediately.

Evaluating Client Response: Postprocedure client and family support in dealing with the results is provided.

■ Oxytocin Challenge Test

Objective Data: Abnormal fetal findings or abnormal or difficult to analyze maternal laboratory findings, particularly estriol levels.

Assessment: The oxytocin challenge test is used to evaluate clients with chronic placental insufficiency or those mothers with abnormal estriol levels. The results indicate those fetuses at risk for intrauterine asphyxia and thus allow for appropriate preventive interventions. OCT is contraindicated in mothers with third trimester bleeding, previous classical cesarean section, or in whom the risk of premature labor outweighs the benefits of this procedure.

Nursing Interventions: Client education includes an explanation of the procedure. Client support for the diagnostic process is provided. Clients are advised to eat before the procedure to avoid interference from bowel sounds. The client empties her bladder before the procedure. During the procedure, the nurse monitors fetal response and oxytocin administration and provides emotional support for the mother.

Description of the Procedure: OCT is performed with inpatients and outpatients. Delivery room facilities must be available close by. The client assumes a semifowler's position. Baseline measurements, including blood pressure, fetal heart rate and activity, and uterine contractions are obtained for 15 minutes. An ultrasonic or phototransducer is placed over the clearest area of fetal heart tones to record the fetal heart rate. A pressure transducer is placed over the fundus to record uterine contractions. If the client has, within 10 minutes, three good quality spontaneous contractions that last 40–60 seconds each, oxytocin is not administered. Otherwise, an IV infusion of 5% dextrose in water is started. Oxytocin solution is then administered piggyback, commonly using an infusion pump, and titrated at 10–20 minute intervals until the client has three good quality uterine contractions in 10 minutes. The maximum amount of oxytocin administered is approximately 20 mU/min. The test is completed when the criteria are met, or when there are three repetitive late decelerations regardless of the frequency of uterine contractions. OCT may require up to $2\frac{1}{2}$ hours to complete. The results are available immediately.

Evaluating Client Response: The mother is monitored until uterine contractions wane and return to the baseline. The fetal heart rate is also monitored. After determination that the results are negative, the client goes home. Client and family support in dealing with the results is provided.

PRENATAL TESTING

- **Chorionic Villi Sampling**
- **Amniocentesis**
- **Fetoscopy**

Clients whose family history includes a genetic disorder may want to determine the presence or absence of such a disorder on a prenatal basis. The family and pregnant client undergoing these procedures need much support in dealing with the test and the results. A specific consent form is required for these procedures.

Nursing Diagnoses for clients undergoing prenatal testing include:

- Alteration in comfort related to procedure
- Anxiety related to procedure
- Knowledge deficit related to diagnostic process
- Potential for pregnancy complications related to procedure

Chorionic Villi Sampling

Subjective Data: A family history suggestive of genetic or fetal disorder.

Objective Data: This test is performed during the first trimester of pregnancy.

Assessment: Chorionic villi sampling is a relatively new procedure that is the focus of much research. It is performed in the first trimester. The fetus is evaluated for chromosomal or genetic abnormality, hereditary metabolic disorder, or anatomical disorder. Preliminary evidence indicates safety for mother and fetus. Potential risks include accidental abortion, infection, and bleeding. The discomfort for the mother is said to be similar to that associated with a Pap smear.

Nursing Interventions: Client education includes an explanation of the procedure. The stage of pregnancy is established. The time required to complete genetic analysis is explained to client and family. If present during the procedure, the nurse provides emotional support, helps the client maintain a still position, and provides technical assistance as needed.

Description of the Procedure: Chorionic villi sampling is performed with inpatients and outpatients. Privacy is provided. The client assumes a supine position. A cannula, 17 cm long and 1.5 mm in diameter, is attached to an obturator and inserted via the cervix. Using ultrasound as a guide, the cannula is rotated to the site of the developing placenta. The obturator is replaced with a 20-ml syringe and 3–10 ml suction is applied. In order to minimize infection, the entire cannula is withdrawn with the suction still applied. From one to three samples are obtained from each client. Some Rh-negative mothers receive Rho-GAM. The procedure is completed in approximately 5 minutes. Clients are discharged soon after, as no cervical dilation has occurred. Clients undergo ultrasound in 2–4 days to affirm continued fetal viability. Genetic determination requires 3–5 weeks to complete.

Evaluating Client Response: Following the procedure, the client is monitored for signs of bleeding. Clients are sent home shortly after the procedure is completed. Client and family support in waiting for and dealing with the results is provided.

■ Amniocentesis (Amniotic Fluid Analysis)

Subjective Data: The family history is suggestive of genetic or fetal disorder.

Objective Data: This test is performed when a pregnancy is at least of 14 weeks duration. Mothers older than 35–40 undergo this procedure.

Assessment: Amniocentesis involves percutaneous removal of amniotic fluid and is performed after the fourteenth week of pregnancy. The major use of amniocentesis is for DNA analysis using recombinant DNA techniques. The fetus is evaluated for chromosomal or genetic abnormality, hereditary metabolic disorder, or anatomical disorder. Fetal maturity, blood group type, Rh factor, and sex can also be determined. The amniotic fluid is also analyzed.

Normal Values:

L/S ratio: > 2:1; diabetic mothers: 3:1 at 35 weeks.
Creatinine: > 2 mg/100 ml at 36 weeks.
Bilirubin: <0.01.
Cytology: 20% of fetal sebaceous gland cells stain orange at 35 or more weeks.

Nursing Interventions: Client education includes an explanation of the procedure. The client is prepared for uterine contractions during the procedure. The time required to complete genetic analysis is discussed with client and family. The mother's Rh type may need to be determined. If present during the procedure, the nurse monitors mothers and fetus, provides emotional support, and also provides technical assistance.

Description of the Procedure: Amniocentesis is performed with inpatients and outpatients. Privacy is provided. The client assumes a supine position and baseline vital signs and fetal heart rate are determined. The entry site is located and prepared. Ultrasound is used as a guide in locating and avoiding the placenta. A small gauge needle is inserted percutaneously. The needle is so small most clients report no discomfort associated with the needle itself. Many clients do, however, experience a strong uterine contraction at the time of insertion. Approximately 15 cc of amniotic fluid are removed. The needle is withdrawn and a dressing is applied to the entry site. Some Rh-negative mothers receive Rho-GAM. The procedure is completed in approximately 30 minutes. Fluid analysis is available in a few days, although genetic determination requires 3–5 weeks.

Evaluating Client Response: Following the procedure, the fetal heart rate is monitored for at least 30 minutes. The mother is monitored for elevation in temperature or bleeding at the entry site. The client is told to report any unusual fetal hyperactivity or lack of movement, vaginal discharge, uterine contractions, abdominal pain or fever, and chills. Client and family support in waiting for and dealing with the results is provided.

■ Fetoscopy

Subjective Data: A family history suggestive of genetic or fetal disorder.

Objective Data: This test is performed when a pregnancy is at least of 18 weeks duration.

Assessment: Fetoscopy, via the birth canal and membranes, is a relatively new procedure used to determine fetal disorders. Fetoscopy is performed to determine the appropriate spot for sampling fetal blood or tissue and for direct visualization of the fetus. This procedure is performed after at least 18 weeks of gestation. Fetoscopy permits detection of disorders that cannot be diagnosed by ultrasound or amniotic fluid analysis, such as the hematologic disorders of hemophilia or beta thalassemia. Fetoscopy is also used to diagnose potentially lethal syndromes that involve skin abnormalities. Fetoscopy does carry risk for the fetus.

Nursing Interventions: Client education includes an explanation of the procedure. Emotional support is provided for the client and family as they explore the risks and benefits of this procedure. Provisions are made for the client to be near the hospital for 2 days following this procedure. The client may be NPO prior to the procedure and may receive IV sedation, often Valium. Antibiotic therapy may be instituted to prevent infection.

Description of the Procedure: Fetoscopy is performed with inpatients and outpatients. The client is supine on the examining table and local anesthetic is administered. The fetoscope, 15 cm long with an outside diameter of 1.7 mm, is inserted through the membranes and guided by ultrasound. After visualization and tissue sampling, the fetoscope is withdrawn. Fetoscopy takes 1–2 hours to complete. The results are available following interpretation.

Evaluating Client Response: Postprocedure client evaluation includes monitoring of vital signs and fetal heart rate for approximately 6 hours. After that, if the mother and fetus are stable, the client leaves the hospital but is told to stay nearby for 2 days. If there is no evidence of fetal distress or spontaneous abortion, the client is free to resume her normal life style. Client and family support in dealing with the procedure and results is provided.

References

GENERAL REFERENCES

Barber TC, Langfitt DE: Teaching the Medical Surgical Patient. Bowie, Maryland, Robert J Brady, 1983

Bloomfield JA: Introduction to Organ Imaging. New York, Medical Examination Publishing, 1984

Brunner LS, Suddarth DS: Textbook of Medical–Surgical Nursing. Philadelphia, JB Lippincott, 1984

Carpenito LJ: Nursing Diagnosis: Application to Clinical Practice. New York, JB Lippincott, 1983

Droske SC, Francis SA: Pediatric Diagnostic Procedures. New York, John Wiley, 1981

Fischbach FT: A Manual of Laboratory Diagnostic Tests, 2nd ed. Philadelphia, JB Lippincott, 1984

Freimarck RT: Attentive patient care can improve DSA quality. Diag Imag p. 48, 1983

Goldberg BB, Wells PNT, eds: Ultrasound in Clinical Diagnosis. New York, Churchill Livingstone, 1983

Gilman AF, Goodman LS, Rall TW, Murad F, eds: Goodman and Gilman's The Pharmacologic Basis of Therapeutics. New York, Macmillan, 1985

Grant EG, Earll J, Richardson JD, Dunne A: High-resolution real-time sonography. Med Clin N Am 68:1609, 1984

Haughey CW: What to say. . .and do. . .when your patient asks about CT scans. Nursing 11:72, 1981

Jaffe MS, Skidmore LC: Diagnostic and Laboratory Tests for Clinical Use. Bowie, Maryland, Robert J Brady, 1984

Katzen BT: Peripheral, abdominal and interventional applications of digital subtraction angiography. Radiol Clin N Am 23:227, 1985

Lamb KJ: Laboratory Tests for Clinical Nursing. Bowie, Maryland, Robert J Brady, 1984

Lee JKJ, Sagel SS, Stanley RJ, eds: Computed Body Tomography. New York, Raven, 1983

Lengel NL: Handbook of Nursing Diagnosis. Bowie, Maryland, Robert J Brady, 1982

Ovitt TW, Newell JD: Digital subtraction angiography: Technology, equipment and techniques. Radiol Clin N Am 23:177, 1985

Parishter DM, Modec MT, Borkowski GP, Weinstein MA, Zeman RK: Magnetic resonance: Principles and applications. Med Clin N Am 68:1393, 1984

Phipps WJ, Long BC, Woods NF: Medical-Surgical Nursing: Concepts and Clinical Practice. St. Louis, CV Mosby, 1983

CHAPTER 2

Bastarache MM, Guica J, Horowitz LM, Shelley MM: Assessing peripheral vascular disease: Noninvasive testing. Am J Nursing 83:1552, 1983

Brenner ZR, Wood KM: Cardiac radionuclide imaging: Patient education. Dimens Crit Care Nurs 3:172, 1984

Brundage BH, Chomka E: Clinical applications of cardiac CT imaging. Mod Concepts Cardiovasc Dis 54:39, 1985

Fennell P: Renin studies. Personal communication. 1986

Funk M: Diagnosis of right ventricular infarction with right precordial leads. Heart Lung 15:562, 1986

Green SE, Popp RL: Role of echocardiography in diagnosis and management of valvular heart disease. Mod Concept Cardiovasc Dis 50:31, 1981

Haughey CW: Preparing your patient for echocardiography. Nursing 14:68, 1984

Hull R: Current approach to diagnosis of deep vein thrombosis. Mod Concepts Cardiovasc Dis 51:129, 1982

Kempczinski RF, Yao JST: Practical Noninvasive Vascular Diagnosis. Chicago, Year Book Medical Publishers, 1982

Lieberman JM, Botte RE, Nelson AD: MRI of the heart. Radiol Clin N Am 22:847, 1984

Pinsky S et al, eds: Imaging of the Peripheral Vascular System. Orlando, Florida, Grune and Stratton, 1984

Rogers RR: Your patient scheduled for electrophysiology studies. Am J Nursing 86:573, 1986

Saddekni S, Sos TA, Srur M, Cohen DJ: Contrast administration and techniques of digital subtraction angiography performance. Radiol Clin N Am 23:275, 1985

Sridharan MR, Flowers NC: Computerized electrocardiographic analysis. Mod Concept Cardiovasc Dis 53:37, 1984

Tobis, JM, Nalcioglu O, Henry WL: Cardiovascular applications of digital subtraction angiography. Mod Concept Cardiovasc Dis 53:31, 1984

CHAPTER 3

Bennett JA: HTLV-III AIDS link. Am J Nursing 85:1086, 1985

CHAPTER 4

Bartlett JG: Invasive diagnostic techniques in respiratory infections. In Pennington JE, ed, Respiratory Infections: Diagnosis and Management. New York: Raven, 1983

Cohen AM: Magnetic resonance imaging of the thorax. Radiol Clin N Am 22:829, 1984

Newell JD: Evaluation of pulmonary and mediastinal disease. Med Clin N AM 68:1463, 1984

Pond G: Pulmonary digital subtraction angiography. Radiol Clin N Am 23:243, 1985

Viamonte M: Chest roentgenography in adults. In Sackner MA, ed, Diagnostic Techniques in Pulmonary Disease. New York, Marcel Dekker, 1980

Wagner HN, Buchanan JW: Radioactive tracer studies in pulmonary disease. In Sackner MA, ed, Diagnostic Techniques in Pulmonary Disease. New York, Marcel Dekker, 1980

Wanner A: Interpretation of pulmonary function tests. In Sackner MA, ed, Diagnostic Techniques in Pulmonary Disease. New York, Marcel Dekker, 1980

Washington JA: Noninvasive diagnostic techniques for lower respiratory infections. In Pennington JE, ed, Respiratory Infections: Diagnosis and Management. New York, Raven, 1983

Wilson JE: Pulmonary angiography. In Sackner MA, ed, Diagnostic Techniques in Pulmonary Disease. New York, Marcel Dekker, 1980

CHAPTER 5

Clark LR, Jaffee MH, Choyke PL, Grant EG, Zeman RK: Pancreatic imaging. Radiol Clin N Am 23:489, 1985

Cox PH, Tjen HSLM: In vivo medical techniques for the evaluation of liver function. In Cox PH, ed, Cholescintigraphy. Boston, Martinus Nijhoff, 1981

Cox PH: Quantitative studies of hepatobiliary transport. In Cox PH, ed, Cholescintigraphy. Boston, Martinus Nijhoff, 1981

Haaga JR: Magnetic resonance imaging of the pancreas. Radiol Clin N Am 22:869, 1984

Helms CA, Katzberg RW, Dolwick MF, eds: Internal Derangements of the Temporomandibular Joint. San Francisco, Radiology Research and Education Foundation, 1983

Jaffee MH, Goldstein HA, Zeman RK, Choyke PL: Noninvasive imaging of the gastrointestinal tract. Med Clin N Am 68:1515, 1984

Parishter DM, Modic MT, Borkowshi GP, Weinstein MA, Zeman RK: Magnetic resonance imaging: Principles and applications. Med Clin N Am 68:1393, 1984

Ravenscroft MM, Swan CHJ: Gastrointestinal Endoscopy and Related Procedures. Baltimore, Williams and Wilkins, 1984

Sleisenger MH, Fordtran JS: Gastrointestinal Disease: Pathology, Diagnosis, Management. Philadelphia, WB Saunders, 1983

Spiro HM: Clinical Gastroenterology, 3rd ed. New York, Macmillan, 1983

Wilson C: Diagnostic work-up for inflammatory bowel disease. Nurs Clin N Am 19:51, 1984

Zeman RK, Jaffee MH, Grant EG, Richardson JD, Clark LR, Choyke PL, Paushter DM: Imaging of the liver, biliary tract and pancreas. Med Clin N Am 68:1535, 1984

Zeman RK, Paushter DM, Schiebler ML, Choyke PL, Jaffee MH, Clark LR: Hepatic imaging: Current status. Radiol Clin N Am 23:473, 1985

CHAPTER 6

Choyke PL, Meranze S, Pahira JJ, Jaffee MH, Grant EG, Zeman RK: Imaging of urinary tract disease: Current approaches. Med Clin N Am 68:1565, 1984

Hillman BJ: Digital radiology of the kidney. Radiol Clin N Am 23:211, 1985

Rifkin MD: Diagnostic Imaging of the Lower Genitourinary Tract. New York, Raven, 1985

CHAPTER 7

Brower AC: The radiologic approach to arthritis. Med Clin N Am 68:1593, 1984
Burgess KE: Cerebral depressants. Nursing 15:47, 1985
Bydder GM: Magnetic resonance imaging of the brain. Radiol Clin N Am 22:779, 1984
Cohen RA, Kaufman RA, Myers PA, Towbin RB: Cranial computerized tomography in the abused child with head injury. Am J Roentgenology 146:97, 1986
Conway-Rutkowski BL: Carini and Owens Neurological and Neurosurgical Nursing, 8th ed. St Louis, CV Mosby, 1982
Galasko CSB, Weber DA, ed: Radionuclide Scintigraphy in Orthopedics. New York, Churchill Livingstone, 1984
Hani JS, Benson JE, Yoon YS: Magnetic resonance imaging in the spinal column and craniovertebral junction. Radiol Clin N Am 22:805, 1984
Kaplan FS: Osteoporosis. Clin Symp 35:15, 1983
Parishter DM, Modic MT, Masaryk TJ: Magnetic resonance imaging of the spine: Applications and limitations. Radiol Clin N Am 23:55, 1985
Ruby EB: Advanced Neurological and Neurosurgical Nursing. St Louis, CV Mosby, 1984
Schellinger D: The low back pain syndrome. Med Clin N Am 68:1631, 1984
Scott JA, Rosenthal DI, Brady TJ: The evaluation of musculoskeletal disease with magnetic resonance imaging. Radiol Clin N Am 22:917, 1984
Seeger JF, Carmody BS: Digital subtraction angiography of the arteries of the head and neck. Radiol Clin N Am 23:178, 1985
Toole JF: Cerebrovascular Disorders, 3rd ed. New York, Raven, 1984
Vogt G, Miller M, Eslver M: Mosby's Manual of Neurological Care. St. Louis, CV Mosby, 1985

CHAPTER 8

Becker SC: The Optics of gonioscopy. In Duane TD, ed, Clinical Ophthalmology. New York, Harper and Row, 1984
Behrendt T: Fluorescein angiography. In Duane TD, ed, Clinical Ophthalmology. New York, Harper and Row, 1984
Behrendt T: Ophthalmoscopy and the normal fundus. In Duane TD, ed, Clinical Ophthalmology. New York, Harper and Row, 1984
Dawson E, ed: The Eye. New York, Academic, 1984
Green D: Laser devices in measuring visual acuity. In Duane TD, ed, Clinical Ophthalmology. New York, Harper and Row, 1984
Guyton DL: Automated clinical refraction. In Duane TD, ed, Clinical Ophthalmology. New York, Harper and Row, 1984

Leutwein K, Lettman, H: The fundus camera. In Duane TD, ed, Clinical Ophthalmology. New York, Harper and Row, 1984

Lichter PR: Gonioscopy. In Duane TD, ed, Clinical Ophthalmology. New York, Harper and Row, 1984

Mohrman R: the Keratometer. In Duane TD, ed, Clinical Ophthalmology. New York, Harper and Row, 1984

Northern JL, ed: Hearing Disorders, 2 ed. Boston, Little Brown and Co, 1984

Parks MM: Sensory tests. In Duane TD, ed, Clinical Ophthalmology. New York, Harper and Row, 1984

Safir A: Retinoscopy. In Duane TD, ed, Clinical Ophthalmology. New York, Harper and Row, 1984

Weinstein GW: Clinical visual electrophysiology. In Duane TD, ed, Clinical Ophthalmology. New York, Harper and Row, 1984

CHAPTER 9

Bobak IM, Jensen MD: Essentials of Maternity Nursing. St Louis, CV Mosby, 1984

Grant EG, Earll J, Richardson JD, Dunne A: High-resolution real-time sonography. Med Clin N Am 68:1609, 1984

Parishter DM, Modec MT, Borkowski GP, Weinstein MA, Zeeman RK: Magnetic resonance: Principles and applications. Med Clin N Am 68:1393, 1984

Olds SB, London ML, Ladewig PA, Davidson SV: Obstetric Nursing. Menlo Park, Addison-Wesley, 1980

Ostchega Y, Culnane M: Tumor markers. Nursing 15:49, 1985

Ravenscroft MM, Swan CHJ: Gastrointestinal Endoscopy and Related Procedures. Baltimore, Williams and Wilkins, 1984

Richardson JD, Cigtay OS, Grant EG, Wang PC: Imaging of the breast. Med Clin N Am 68:1481, 1984

CHAPTER 10

Beeson D, Douglas R: Prenatal diagnosis of fetal disorders, Part 1: Technological capabilities. Birth 10:227, 1983

Ward RHT, Modell B, Petrou M, Karagozlu V, Douratsos E: Method of sampling chorionic villi in 1st trimester of pregnancy under guidance of real time ultrasound. Br Med J 286:1542, 1983

Index

Abdominal x-rays, 149
Acetaminophen, 204
Acetoacetate, 111
Acid phosphatase, 267
Acid-fast bacilli stain (AFB), 81
ACTH stimulation test, 128–130
Activated partial thromboplastin time (APTT), 66
Afterimage test, 250
Air encephalography, 246
Albumin, 171
Albumin-globulin ratio (A/G ratio), 117
Alcohol ethanol, 203
Aldolase, 111
Aldosterone, 171
Alkaline phosphatase (ALP), 111
Allergic response skin test, 85
Alpha-1-antitrypsin, 79
Alphafetoprotein, (AFP), 267
Amikacin, 66
Ammonia (NH_3), 111
Amniocentesis, 295–296
Amoxicillin, 67
Ampicillin, 67
Amylase, 112
Androstanedione, 267
Angiography
  fluid volume impairments, 194–195
  tissue perfusion alteration, 52–53
  mobility impairment, 243–244
  nutrition, metabolism, and elimination alteration, 158–159
Anorectal motility, 122–123
Anoscopy, 163–164
Antinuclear antibodies (ANA), 202
Aortography, 52
Arterial blood gases (ABG), 79
Arteriography, 52
Arthrocentesis, 228–229
Arthrography, 241–242
Arthroscopy, 226–227
Audiogram, 251–252
Audiology testing, 251–252

Auditory brainstem response (ABR), 210–211
Automated clinical refractor test, 249
Avionics, 23

Bagoline striated glasses test, 249
Band cells, 62
Barbiturate, 203
Barium enema (BE), 155–157
Barium swallow, 154–155
Basophils, 62
Bence-Jones protein, 171
Bernstein test, 123–124
bG chemstrip capillary, 114
Bile acid breath test, 132
Bilirubin, 112
Biopsy
 arthrocentesis, 228–229
 bone marrow, 75
 breast, 282
 definition of, 11
 endometrial smear, 282
 fluid volume impairment, 199
 gas exchange impairment, 106
 liver, 166
 lung, 107
 mobility impairment, 228–232
 muscle, 230–231
 nerve, 231
 nutrition, metabolism, and elimination alterations, 166–168
 paracentesis, 167
 percutaneous renal, 199–200
 sexual dysfunction, 278–279, 282–283
 transiliac bone, 229–230
 transtrachial aspiration, 106
Bithermal caloric test, 263–264
Blastomycosis skin test, 83
Bleeding time, 60
Blood count, complete, 61
Blood culture, 63
Blood typing, 60
Blood urea nitrogen (BUN), 170
Bone density test, 217
Bone marrow biopsy, 75
Bone marrow scan, 71
Bone scan, 216
Brain scan, 217–218
Breast biopsy, 282
Breast self-examination, 265–266
Breath test
 bile acid, bilary stage, 132–133
 hydrogen, 131–132
 nutrition, metabolism, and elimination alterations, 131–133
 triolein, 132
Bronchial provocation test, 86–89
Bronchography, 102–103
Bronchoscopy, 104
Brucellosis skin test, 83
BVAT microprocessor test, 249

C-peptide, 113
C-reactive protein, (CRP), 63
Cadmium, 203
Calcitonin, 112
Calcium, 172
Caloric stimulation test, 263
Captopril, 19
Carbamazepine, 203
Carbenicillin, 67
Carbon dioxide (CO_2), 80
Carbon monoxide, 203
Carcinoembryonic antigen (CEA), 112
Cardiac catheterization, 53–55
Cardiac mapping, 25
Carotene, 112
Carotid angiography, 243–244
Cefamandole, 67
Cefazolin, 67
Cefoxitin, 67
Cephalexin, 67
Cephalothin, 67
Cephradine, 67
Cerebral arterography, 243–244
Cerebral blood flow study, 218–219
Cervical biopsy, 278–279
Cervical scrape, 266
Chest x-rays, 45, 95–97

Chloramphenicol, 67
Chlordiazepoxide, 203
Chloride, 172
Chloroquine, 67
Chlorpromazine, 203
Cholecystokinin test (CCK), 125–126
Cholescintigraphy, 144
Cholesterol, 17
Cholinesterase RBC, 202
Chorionic villi sampling, 294–295
Cimetidine, 119
Cisternal puncture, 238–239
Cisternal scan, 220–221
Clindamycin, 67
Clonazepam, 204
Cloxacillin, 67
Coagulation factor concentration test, 61
Coagulation time (Lee-White clotting time), 61
Coccidiodomycosis skin test, 83
Cold aglutinins, 80
Cold spot scan, 35
Colonoscopy, 161–162
Color plates test, 249
Colpomicroscopy, 278–279
Colposcopy, 278–279
Complement fixation flocculation, 270
Complement total, 61
Complete blood count, (CBC), 61
Computed tomography,
  definition of, 4, 6
  fluid volume impairment, 186–187
  gas exchange impairment, 98–99
  mobility impairment, 224–225
  nutrition, metabolism, and elimination alterations, 151–152
  sexual dysfunction, 276–277
  tissue perfusion alteration examination, 46–47
Computed tomography metrizamide myelography (CTMM), 224–225
Computer assisted myelography (CAM), 224–225
Contrast studies
  air encephalography, 246
  angiography, 52–53
  arthrography, 241–242
  bronchography, 102–103
  carotid angiography, 243–244
  coronary angiography, 53–55
  cystourethrogram, 191–192
  definition of, 8–11
  digital subtraction angiography. *See* Digital subtraction angiography
  family process alterations, 290–291
  fluid volume impairment, 188–195
  gas exchange impairment, 100–103
  hysterosalpingogram, 290–291
  infusion drip pyelogram, 189–190
  intravenous urogram, 188–189
  lower GI series, 155–157
  mobility impairment, 241–246
  myelography, 245–246
  nutrition, metabolism, and elimination alterations, 153–159
  percutaneous transhepatic cholangiography, 157–158
  pulmonary angiography, 101–102
  renal angiogram, 194–195
  retrograde pyelogram, 190–191
  retrograde urethrogram, 192–193
  temporomandibular joint arthrography, 153–154
  tissue perfusion alteration examination, 50–55
  upper gastrointestinal study, 154
  venography, 50–51
  vesiculogram, 291
Coomb's test (DAGT, IAGT), 61
Copper, 113
Coronary angiography, 53–55
Cortisol level, 128–130
Creatinine, 173
Creatinine clearance, 173
Creatinine photokinase (CPK), 15
Crossmatching, 60
CT. *See* Computed tomography
Culdoscopy, 280–281
Cyclosporine, 67
Cystograms, 189–190
Cystometrography, 179–180

Cystoscopy, 196–197
Cystourethrogram, 191–192
Cytology, 81

D-Xylose absorption-excretion test, 125
D-Xylose tolerance test, 125
Dental x-rays, 149
Desipramine, 204
Dexamethasone suppression test, 128–130
Diagnex blue, 120–121
Diazepam, 204
Diazoxide, 19
Dick skin test, 83
Dicloxacillin, 67
Differential (white blood cells), 62
Difficult speech audiometry, 252
Diffusion tests, 86–89
Digital subtraction angiography (DSA)
  definition of, 10
  fluid volume impairment, 193–194
  gas exchange impairment, 100–101
  mobility impairment, 242–243
  tissue perfusion alterations, 51–52
Digitoxin, 19
Digoxin, 19
Diphenhydramine, 204
Direct visualization
  anoscopy, 163–164
  colonoscopy, 161–162
  colposcopy, 278–279
  culdoscopy, 280–281
  endoscopic retrograde cholangiopancreaticography, 164–165
  fluid volume impairment, 196–198
  gas exchange impairment, 104–105
  hysteroscopy, 279
  laparoscopy, 280
  mobility impairment, 226–227
  nutrition, metabolism, and elimination alterations, 160–165
  percutaneous nephroscopy, 197–198
  sexual dysfunction, 278–281
  upper gastrointestinal fiberoscopy, 160
  urethroscopy, 196–197
Direct visualization of the eye
  gonioscopy, 255
  ophthalmoscopy, 253–254
DISIDA scan, 144
Disopyramide, 19
Diuretic radionuclide urogram, 182
Doppler ultrasonography
  definition, 2
  examination, 29–30
  imaging, 29–30
Doxepin, 204
Doxycycline, 67
Drug levels
  gas exchange impairment, 80
  injury or infection potential, 66–68
  mobility impairment, 203–204
  nutrition, metabolism, and elimination alterations, 119
  tissue perfusion alterations, for, 19–20
DSA. *See* Digital subtraction angiography
Dual photon absorptiometry, 217

ECG. *See* Electrocardiography
Echocardiography, 28
Ectopic mucosa scan, 141–142
EKG. *See* Electrocardiography
Electrical activity measurement
  electrocardiography, 21–26
  electroencephalography, 210–211
  electromyography, 209–210
  electronystagmography, 258–259
  electroretinography, 257–258
  mobility impairment, 209–211
  sensory input alterations, 257–259
Electrocardiography, 21
  electrophysiology studies, 25–26
  exercise testing, 23–24
  Holter monitoring, 23
  tissue perfusion alterations, 21–26
  twelve lead, 21–22

Electroencephalography, 210–211
Electrolytes, 172–173
Electromyography, 209–210
Electronystagmography (ENG), 258
Electro-oculography (EOG), 257–258
Electrophysiology studies, 25–26
Electroretinography (ERG), 257
EMI. *See* Computed tomography
Endocervical smear, 266
Endometrial smear, 282–283
Endoscopic retrograde cholangiopancreaticography (ERCP), 164–165
Endoscopy, 160–161
Enteroclysis, 154–155
Eosinophils, 62
EPS. *See* Electrophysiology studies
Equilibrium study, 27
Erthryocyte sedimentation rate (ESR), 63
Erythrocyte fragility, 15
Erythromycin, 67
Erythroprotein, 15
Esophageal motility, 122–123
Esophageal scan, 139
Esophagoscopy, 160–161
Estradiol, 268
Estriol, 268
Estrogens, 268
Estrone, 268
Ethambutol, 80
Ethosuximide, 204
Evoked potential studies, 210–211
Excretory urogram, 188–189
Exercise testing
  electrocardiography, 23–24
  thallium, 35
Expiratory force test, 88
Expiratory reserve volume test, 88

Fecal culture, 113
Fecal fat/mucus/pus, 113
Ferritin, 15
Fertility tests
  Rubin's test, 288–289
  seminal fluid analysis, 286–287
  Sims-Huhner test, 287–288
  testicular scan, 287
Fetal acceleration determination, 292
Fetal testing
  nonstress testing, 292
  oxytocin challenge test, 293
Fetoscopy, 296–297
Fibrin degradation products (FDP), 64
Fibrin split products (FSP), 63
Fibrinogen, 64
Fibrinopeptide A (FPA), 64
First transit study, 37
Fishberg concentration test, 173
Flow volume loop, 89
Floxacillin, 67
Flucytosine, 67
Fluorescein angiography, 262
Fluorescent antibody, 270
Fluorescent antibody test, 65
Folate, 113
Folic acid, 15, 113
Follicle stimulating hormone (FSH), 268
Forced endexpiratory flow test, 88
Forced expiratory flow test, 88
Forced expiratory volume test, 87
Forced inspiration flow test, 88
Forced inspiratory capacity test, 88
Forced midexpiratory flow test, 88
Forced vital capacity test, 87
Free thyroxine (FT4), 118
Free triiodothyronine (FT3), 118
Frei skin test, 83
FTA-ABS, 270
Functional residual capacity test, 89
Furosemide, 173

Galactose tolerance test, 124–125
Galactose-1-phosphate uridyl transferase, 113
Gall bladder scan, 144
Gallium scan, 71–72
Gastric analysis, 120–121
Gastric emptying scan, 140–141

Gastrin, 114
Gastroesophageal reflux scan, 140
Gastroscopy, 160–161
Gated blood pool studies, 37
Gentamycin, 67
Glucagon, 114
Glucose fasting, 114
Glucose tolerance test, 124–125
Glucose-6-phosphate dehydrogenase (GPD), 16
Glutathione reductase (GR), 16
Glycosylate hemoglobin, 115
Gonioscopy, 255
Gonorrhea culture, 269
Gram stain, 81
Growth hormone, 114
Guaiac, 114
Guinidine, 20

Haloperidol, 204
Heaf gun skin test, 84
Heinz bodies, 16
Hemagglutination, 270
Hemagglutination inhibition (HI, HAI), 66
Hematocrit (HCT), 18
Hemoglobin (Hgb), 18
Hemoglobin A1c, 115
Hemoglobin electrophoresis, 16
Hemoglobin S (Hgb S), 18
Hepatitis antigen (HAA, HB), 115
Heterophile antibody test, 65
Hexsaminidase, 115
Hexsaminidase A, 115
Hgb S, 18
Histoplasmosis skin test, 83
HLA-B27 HLA-TMO, 202
Holter monitoring electrocardiography, 23
Hot spot imaging, 36
Human chorionic gonadotropin (HCG), 269
Human immunodeficiency virus (HIV), 64
Hydatid skin test, 83
Hydralazine, 19
Hydrogen breath test, 131–132
Hydroxyproline, 202
Hysterosalpingogram, 290–291
Hysteroscopy, 279

IgA, 64
IgE, 64
IgG, 64
IgM, 64
Imipramine, 204
Immunoglobulins, 64
Impedance audiometry, 251–252
Impedance plethysmography, 32
In vivo scintigraphy, 143–144
In vivo studies, 41–42
Indirect ophthalmoscopy, 254
Indocyanine green, 115
Indomethacin, 204
Infarct imaging scintigraphy, 36–37
Infectious disease skin test, 82
Infusion drip pyelogram, 189–190
Inorganic phosphate, 116
Inspiratory capacity test, 88
Inspiratory force test, 88
Insulin tolerance test, 126–127
Intraarterial angiography, 10
Intravenous pyelography (IVP), 188–189
Intravenous urogram (IVU), 188–189
Iodine-125-fibrinogen leg scintigraphy, 40
Iodine-125-fibrinogen uptake test, 39
Iontophoresis sweat test, 128
Iron, 16
Isocitric dehydrogenase, 115
Isoenzyme, 115

Keratometer measurement, 254
Ketone bodies, 115
Kidney scan, 181–182
Kidney ureter bladder films (KUB), 185

Labetolol, 19
Laboratory tests
  fluid volume impairment, 171–174
  gas exchange impairment, 79–80
  injury or infection potential, 60–66
  mobility impairment, 202–203
  nutrition, metabolism, and elimination alterations, 111–119
  sexual dysfunction, 267–270
  tissue perfusion alterations, 15–19
Lactic acid dehydrogenase (LDH), 115
  isoenzymes, 17
Lactose tolerance test, 124–125
Laminography, 261
Lancaster projector test, 249
Laparoscopy, 280
Lateral cervical puncture, 237–238
Latex fixation, 203
Lead, 204
Lee-White clotting time, 61
Letter chart test, 249
Leucine aminopeptidase, 116
Leukocyte alkaline phosphatase, 64
Lidocaine, 19
Lipase, 116
Lipids total, 17
Lithium, 204
Liver biopsy, 166
Liver–spleen scan, 145
Lorcainide, 19
Lower GI series, 155–157
Lumbar puncture (LP), 233
Lumbar sympathetic block, 48–49
Lung biopsy, 107
Lung scan, 92–93
Luteinizing hormone (LH), 269
Lymphangiography, 73–74
Lymphocytes, 63
Lysozyme, 65

M Mode ultrasonography, 2
Magnesium, 116, 172
Magnetic resonance imaging
  definition of, 4
  fluid volume impairment, 177
  gas exchange impairment, 91
  mobility impairment, 213–214
  nutrition, metabolism, and elimination, 136–137
  sexual dysfunction, 273
  tissue perfusion alteration examination, 34
Major amblyscope test, 250
Mammography, 274–275
Manganese, 116
Manometric test, 233–235
Mantoux skin test, 84
Maximal voluntary ventilation, 88
Mean corpuscular hemoglobin (MCH), 18
Mean corpuscular hemoglobin concentration (MCHC), 18
Mean corpuscular volume (MCV), 19
Measurement of electrical activity. *See* Electrical activity measurement
Meckel's scan, 141–142
Meperidine, 204
Methacycline, 67
Methanol, 204
Methicillin, 67
Methotrexate, 67
Methsuximide, 204
Metoprolol, 19
Metronidazole, 119
Mexiletine, 19
Microhematocrit, 18
Mictuariting cystourethrogram (MCU), 191–192
Minocycline, 67
Minute respiratory volume test, 89
Modified Schwabach test, 251
Monocytes, 63
Mononucleosis tests, 65
Motility and challenge tests
  Bernstein test, 123–124
  cortisol level, 128–130
  d-Xylose absorption-excretion test, 125

Motility and challenge tests *(cont.)*
d-Xylose tolerance test, 125
glucose tolerance test, 124–125
insulin tolerance test, 126–127
motility tests, 122–123
pancreatic secretion test, 125–126
sweat electrolyte test, 128
thyrotropin releasing hormone stimulation, 130
tolbutamide tolerance test, 127–128
Motility tests, 122
MRI. *See* Magnetic resonance imaging
MUGA scan, 37
Mumps skin test, 84
Muramidase, 65
Muscle biopsy, 230–231
Myelography, 245–246
Myocardial imaging, 36

Naproxen, 204
Needle aspiration of lung, 107–108
Neonatal thyroptropin stimulating hormone, 118
Nephroscopy, 196–197
Nephrotomogram, 189–190
Nerve biopsy, 231
Nerve conduction study, 209–210
Netilmicin, 67
Neutrophils, 62
Nitrazepam, 204
Nitroglycerine, 19
Nonimaging scintigraphy, 143–144
Nonstress testing (NST), 292
Norland-Cameron single photon absorptiometry, 217
Nortriptyline, 204
Nuclear angiocardiography, 37–38
Nuclear medicine
definition, 4–5

Ocular plethysmography (OPG), 207–208
Ocular pneumoplethysmography (OPG-GEE), 207–208
Oculovestibular reflex test, 263–264
Ophthalmoscopy, 253–254
Original direct ophthalmoscopy, 254
Osmolality, 174
Oxacillin, 67
Oxytocin challenge test, 293

Pancreas scan, 145–146
Pancreatic secretion test, 125–126
Papanicolaou (Pap) smear, 266
Paracentesis, 167
Parathyroid hormone (PTH), 116
Parotid gland scan, 138–139
Peak expiratory flow rate, 88
Pelvic endoscopy, 280–281
Pelvic peritoneoscopy, 280–281
Penicillin G, 67
Pentose tolerance test, 124–125
Percent saturation, 16
Percutaneous nephroscopy, 197–198
Percutaneous renal biopsy, 199–200
Percutaneous transhepatic cholangiography (PTC), 157–158
Perfusion imaging scintigraphy, 35–36
Perfusion scan, 92
Peripheral ultrasonography, 29
Phensuximide, 204
Phenylbutazone, 204
Phenylketonuria (PKU), 202
Phenytoin, 204
Phlebogram, 50
Phonocardiography, 27
Phonoangiography, 27
Phospholipids LDH isoenzymes, 17
Phosphorous (PO_4), 116
Phosphorus, 172
Photon absorptiometry, 217
Photoplethysmography, 32–33
P-K test, 287–288
Pindolol, 20
Placental hormone test, 269
Platelet adhesion, 65

Platelet aggregation, 65
Platelet volume, 65
Platelets, 62
Plethysmography
  impedance, 32–33
  photoplethysmography, 32–33
  strain gauge, 31–32
  tissue perfusion alterations, 31–33
Pleural biopsy, 107–108
Pneumoencephalography, 246
Potassium, 17, 172
Potassium hydroxide wet mount, 81
Pregnancy test, 269
Pregnanediol, 269
Pregnanetriol, 116
Prenatal testing
  amniocentesis, 295–296
  chorionic villi sampling, 294–295
  fetoscopy, 296–297
Primidone, 204
Procainamide, 20
Proctoscopy, 163–164
Prolactin, 117
Propanolol, 20
Porphyrins and porphobilinogens, 116
Prostatic acid phosphate (PAP), 270
Protein total, 117
Protein electrophoresis, 117
Protein-bound iodine (PBI), 118
Prothrombin time, 65
Protriptyline, 204
Pulmonary angiography, 101
Pulmonary function tests (PFT), 86
  diffusion tests, 89
  expiratory force, 88
  expiratory reserve volume (ERV), 88
  flow volume loop (FVL), 89
  forced endexpiratory flow, 88
  forced expiratory flow, 88
  forced expiratory volume (FEV), 87
  forced inspiration flow (FIF), 88
  forced inspiratory volume (FIV), 88
  forced midexpiratory flow, 88
  forced vital capacity (FVC), 87
  functional residual capacity (FRC), 89
  inspiratory capacity (IC), 88
  inspiratory force (IF), 88
  maximal voluntary ventilation (MVV), 88
  minute respiratory volume, 89
  peak expiratory flow rate (PFR, PEFR), 88
  rebreathing, 89
  residual volume (RV), 89
  single breath, 89
  steady-state, 89
  tidal volume (TV), 89
  total lung capacity (TLC), 89
  vital capacity (VC), 87
Pure tone air conduction and bone conduction tests, 252
Pyridostigmine, 204

Quinidine, 20
Queckenstedt test, 235–237

Radioactive gas perfusion tests, 94
Radioactive iodine uptake test, 146–147
Radioactive triolen uptake, 117
Radioimmunoassay allegosorbent (RAST), 80
Radioisotope angiogram, 219–220
Radiology
  abdominal x-rays, 149
  chest x-rays, 45, 95–97
  computed tomography, 98–99. *See also* Computed tomography
  definition of, 5–6
  dental x-rays, 149
  fluid volume impairment, 185
  gas exchange impairment, 95–99
  mobility impairment, 222–223
  sensory input alterations, 261
  sexual dysfunction, 274–278
  sinus x-rays, 95
  tissue perfusion alteration examination, 45
  tomography, 96

Radionuclide angiography, 38–39
Radionuclide cystogram, 183–184
Radionuclide venography, 40–41
Rantidine, 119
RBC indices, 18
Rebreathing test, 89
Rectosigmoidoscopy, 161–162
Red blood cell indices, 18
Red blood cells (RBC), 17
Red filter test, 249
Regional cerebral blood flow study, 218–219
Renal angiogram, 194–195
Renal biopsy, 199–200
Renal scan, 181–182
Renin studies, 56–57
Renne test, 251
Renogram, 182
Residual volume test, 89
Reticulocyte count, 19
Retinol, 112
Retinoscopy, 254
Retrograde pyelogram, 190–191
Retrograde urethrogram, 192–193
Rh factor, 66
Rheumatoid factor (RA factor), 203
RPR, 270
Rubella titer, 66
Rubin's test, 288–289

Salicylate, 204
Salivary gland scan, 138
Schilling test, 43–44
Scintigraphic gastrointestinal bleeding study, 142–143
Scintigraphy
  bone marrow scan, 71
  bone scan, 216
  brain scan, 217–218
  cerebral blood flow study, 218–219
  cisternal scan, 220–221
  definition of, 4–5
  diuretic radionuclide urogram, 182
  ectopic mucosa scan, 141–142
  esophageal scan, 139
  fluid volume impairment, 181–184
  gall bladder scan, 144
  gallium scan, 71–72
  gas exchange impairment, 92–94
  gastric emptying scan, 140–141
  gastroesophageal reflux scan, 140
  in vivo studies, 41–43
  infarct imaging, 36–37
  injury or infection potential, 70–72
  iodine-125–fibrinogen leg, 40
  iodine-125–fibrinogen uptake test, 39
  kidney scan, 181–182
  liver-spleen scan, 145
  mobility impairment, 215–221
  nonimaging, 143–144
  nuclear angiocardiography, 37–38
  nutrition, metabolism, and elimination alterations, 138–144
  pancreas scan, 145–146
  perfusion imaging, 35–36, 92–93
  photon absorptiometry, 217
  radioactive gas perfusion tests, 94
  radioactive iodine uptake test, 146
  radioisotope angiogram, 219–220
  radionuclide angiography, 38–39
  radionuclide cystogram, 183–184
  radionuclide venography, 40–41
  renogram, 182
  salivary gland scan, 138
  Schilling test, 43–44
  scintigraphic gastrointestinal bleeding study, 142–143
  spleen scan, 70
  synovial scan, 215–216
  thyroid scan, 147–149
  ventilation scan, 93–94
Secretin test, 125–126
Semen test, 286–287
Seminal fluid analysis, 286–287
Sensory acuity tests
  audiology tests, 251
  tuning fork tests, 250
  vision tests, 248

Serum angiotensin converting enzyme (SACE), 80
Serum glutamicoxaloacetic transaminase (SGOT), 117
Serum glutamicpyruvic transaminase (SGPT), 118
17 ketosteroids, 269
Shick skin test, 84
Sigmoidoscopy
  flexible, 161–162
  rigid, 163–164
Sims-Huhner test, 287–288
Single breath test, 89
Sinus x-rays, 95
Skeletal survey, 216
Skin tests
  allergic response, 85
  blastomycosis, 83
  brucellosis, 83
  coccidiodomycosis, 83
  dick, 83
  Frei, 83
  gas exchange impairment, 82
  heaf gun, 84
  histoplasmosis, 83
  hydatid, 83
  infectious disease, 82
  mantoux, 84
  mumps, 84
  Shick, 84
  soft chancre, 84
  tine, 84
  toxicoplasmosis, 84
  trichinosis, 84
  tularemia, 84
Slit-lamp ophthalmoscopy, 254
Snellen eye test, 249
Sodium, 173
Soft chancre skin test, 84
Small bowel series, 154–155
Speech discrimination test, 251–252
Speech reception test, 252
Sperm count, 286–287
Spinal dynamics, 235–237
Spinal puncture
  cisternal puncture, 238–239
  lateral cervical puncture, 237–238
  lumbar puncture, 233–235
  spinal dynamics, 235–237
  subdural puncture, 239–240
Spinal tap, 233–235
Spleen scan, 70
Sputum culture, 81
Sputum testing, 80–81
Steady-state test, 89
Strain gauge plethysmography, 31–32
Stress testing, 23
Subdural puncture, 239–240
Sweat electrolyte test, 128
Synovial fluid analysis, 228–229
Synovial scintigraphy, 215–216
Syphilis detection, 270

Technetium scan, 36
Temporomandibular joint (TMJ) arthrography, 153–154
Terbutaline, 80
Testicular scan, 287
Testicular self-examination, 266
Testosterone, 270
Tetracycline, 68
Thallium scan, 35
Theophylline, 80
Thermography, 212
Thoracentesis, 107–108
Thorn test, 128–130
Throat culture, 81
Thrombin clotting time, 66
Thyroglobulin (Tg), 118
Thyroid function tests, 118
Thyroid scan, 147–148
Thyroid stimulating hormone (TSH), 118
Thyrotropin releasing hormone stimulation test, 130
Thyroxine (T4), 118
Thyroxine binding globulin, 118
Tidal volume test, 89
Timolol, 20
Tine skin test, 84

Tobramycin, 68
Tocainide, 20
Tolbutamide, 119
Tolbutamide tolerance test, 127–128
Tomography
  gas exchange impairment, 96
  nutrition, metabolism, and elimination alterations, 149
  sensory input alterations, 261
Tone decay test, 252
Tonometry, 256
Total iron binding capacity (TIBC), 16
Total lung capacity test, 89
Toxicoplasmosis skin test, 84
TP-MHA, 270
Transferrin, 118
Transiliac bone biopsy, 229–230
Transtrachial aspiration, 106
Trichinosis skin test, 84
Triglycerides, 17
Triiodothyronine (T3), 118
Trimethadione, 204
Triolein breath test, 132–133
Triolen 1311 absorption test, 117
Tubal insufflation, 288–289
Tubular reabsorption phosphate (TPR), 119
Tularemia skin test, 84
Tuning fork tests, 250–251
12 lead electrocardiography, 21–22
Two-hour postprandial, 114

Ultrasonography
  definition of, 1–4
  Doppler, 2, 4, 29–30
  echocardiography, 28
  fluid volume impairment, 175–176
  gas exchange impairment, 90
  injury or infection potential, 69
  M mode, 2
  mobility impairment, 205–206
  nutrition, metabolism, and elimination alterations, 134–135
  peripheral, 29
  pulsed Dopplers, 4
  sensory input alterations, 260
  sexual dysfunction, 271–272
  tissue perfusion alteration examination, 29–30
Upper gastrointestinal fiberoscopy, 160
Upper gastrointestinal study (UGI), 154–155
Urethral pressure profile, 179
Urethroscopy, 196–197
Uric acid, 174
Urinalysis, 174
Urine (sugar acetone, AC urine, DU), 114
Urine culture, 174
Urobilinogen, 119
Urodynamic measurements
  cystometrography, 179–180
  urethral pressure profile, 179
  uroflowmetry, 178–179
Uterotubogram, 290–291

Valproic acid, 204
Vancomycin, 68
Vanillylmandelic acid (UMA), 174
VDRL, 270
Vectorgraphic test for suppression, 250
Venography, 50–51
Ventilation scan, 93–94
Ventilatory function tests, 86–89
Ventricular tap, 239–240
Ventriculography, 246
Verapamil, 20
Vesiculogram, 291
Viral antibody test, 66
Vision tests, 248

Visual evoked potential (VEP), 210–211
Vital capacity, 87
Vitamin A, 112
Vitamin B_{12}, 19
Vitamin D and metabolites, 203
Voiding cystourethrogram, 191–192

Weber test, 251
White blood cell count (WBC), 62
Worth 4-dot test, 249

X-ray pelvimetry, 274
X-rays. *See* Radiology